TASTING YOUR
OWN MEDICINE

TASTING YOUR OWN MEDICINE

HOW TO ADVOCATE FOR YOURSELF IN HEALTH CARE SETTINGS

KARAN K. MIRPURI

NEW DEGREE PRESS

COPYRIGHT © 2021 KARAN K. MIRPURI

TASTING YOUR OWN MEDICINE

How to Advocate for Yourself in Health Care Settings

ISBN   978-1-63676-905-9   *Paperback*

978-1-63676-969-1   *Kindle Ebook*

978-1-63730-073-2   *Ebook*

For my Mom and my Dad, whose unconditional love and guidance have helped me embrace my own inner magic.

and

For Rachel (Lava), who welcomed me into a family that inspires me to find the magic in others.

CONTENTS

INTRODUCTION

———

Molly Hottle walked into the hospital one ordinary day, ready for a routine doctor's appointment. As a health care communications professional, the setting was one that felt familiar. Her education had equipped her to understand the complex jargon spoken by health professionals and to help others navigate the intricacies of medical care. However, despite having this reservoir of knowledge, she was unable to advocate for herself when it mattered most.[1]

When she entered the doors of her doctor's office, she was greeted by a medical assistant, who informed her she needed to take a lab test. She didn't know what it was for, but she went along with it, finding it easier to comply than to ask any questions.

"You know how you feel rushed when you go to the doctor's office? Even though you're the patient, it's supposed to be about you and your health. They're speaking a foreign language,

---

[1]   *TEDx Talks,* "Advocate for Your Health | Molly Hottle | TEDxTucson," March 6, 2017, video, 14:56.

you're intimidated, and it just seems easier to go along with things than to ask questions. Sometimes it costs you."[2]

To this day, Molly has no idea what that lab test was for. What she does remember, however, is the two-thousand-dollar bill she received in the mail a few weeks later, one she had to fight for months. According to her health insurance company, the test was not medically necessary. They refused to cover it. In the process of fighting this bill, she repeatedly asked herself why she didn't just ask what the test was for. As she revealed in her TEDx Talk "Advocate for Your Health," it's a question that still plagues her.

"I am a health care communicator. I am getting my master's degree in this very field. This is not supposed to happen to me. But it did."[3]

During her talk, Molly brings up a compelling statistic: annually, more than 250,000 patient deaths are a result of *misdiagnosis.*[4] However, we have absolutely no idea how many deaths occur as a result of *misunderstanding* as a result of miscommunication, a point she highlights through the unfortunate experiences of other medical patients.

One story involved a thirty-year-old woman who ended up undergoing a hysterectomy without knowing her uterus was removed until weeks after the operation when a nurse asked her about the surgery during a follow-up, all because

---

2   Ibid.
3   Ibid.
4   Ibid.

she signed forms filled with language beyond her level of comprehension.[5] Another story, from Anne Fadiman's *The Spirit Catches You and You Fall Down: A Hmong Child, Her American Doctors, and the Collision of Two Cultures* (1997), revealed how the language barrier between a young Hmong girl's parents and her American doctors prevented them from understanding her doctors' recommendations to treat her epilepsy with anti-seizure medication. As a result of the confusion, the doctors never gave the medication to her, leaving the girl in a vegetative coma at the age of four that persisted until she died.[6]

These stories were heartbreaking to listen to, and frankly, quite frustrating. But for some reason, my mind kept drifting back to Molly's personal narrative. As I felt her palpable anger strike me in my core, I wondered how it was possible someone within the system could find themselves in a situation like this. A lot of medical shows (trust me, I've watched many) usually include an episode ridiculing medical professionals who are awful patients and awful parents. Their extensive knowledge of human anatomy and disease makes them overbearing and quick to consider the worst possibilities, much to the annoyance of other doctors. Now seeing an instance where even a health professional was effectively silenced in a medical setting, I wondered: *how is it that our system prevents even the most well-versed individuals from advocating for their health?*

---

5   Ibid.

6   Anne Fadiman, *The Spirit Catches You and You Fall Down: A Hmong Child, Her American Doctors, and the Collision of Two Cultures* (New York: Farrar, Straus and Giroux, 1997).

It's not a secret the field of medicine is difficult to navigate. As a sophomore in college on the premedical track, I still have three more of years of undergraduate education before I embark on four years of medical school. That's not even including the years of residency and fellowship before I can actually become a board-certified physician. But while health professionals undergo a very rigorous educational regimen, the same cannot be said for patients.

Every day, ordinary people are thrust into a totally foreign world where random strangers in white coats and scrub caps are suddenly in control of whether they live or die. The challenge is exacerbated by the complexities of medical language, insurance, and the often consequently overlooked emotional and mental stress. While health classes teach us some basic fundamentals to maintain a healthy lifestyle, such as maintaining a balanced diet, exercising frequently, and minimizing our consumption of substances, we are never formally taught how to interact with our doctors, what kinds of questions to ask, and how to prepare ourselves for potentially life-changing decisions. Additionally, although many education initiatives are in place to increase our accessibility and understanding of valuable health resources, health literacy and numeracy still tends to be low, especially for those with language barriers, limited accessibility to health resources, and a lower socioeconomic status. Studies have also shown such adults with low health literacy and numeracy experience up to four times higher health care costs, 6 percent more hospital visits, and average hospital stays of two days longer.[7]

---

7   Center for Health Care Strategies, "What is Health Literacy?," 2013.

Having had numerous long-term and short-term doctors throughout my life, I have experienced the frustration and anxiety of being a patient multiple times. Despite the more difficult aspects of being a patient, I genuinely loved the opportunities I had to truly communicate with my doctors and understand what was going on with my body and my health. Yes, there were times I wanted to please my doctor and be the best patient I could, but I wouldn't let that stop me from asking them questions to quell my fears or sate my curiosity. While it's easy for us to think being inquisitive about our medical care will make us come off as annoying or bratty, research and conversations with those in the medical industry have changed the way I engage with my care today.

While a certain proverb warns people not to be too inquisitive for their own good, I've found curiosity, in many ways, can actually cure the cat, rather than kill it. The curious patient is one who takes control of their health. They acknowledge the expertise of their medical professionals but are not afraid to ask the questions they need to make informed decisions about their care. Rather than craving the approval of their physician, they crave their guidance and seek opportunities to have conversations and ask for help when needed. Not only do they feel more in control of their care but this active engagement can also potentially facilitate better outcomes.

Through this book, I will try to redefine what constitutes a good patient and simultaneously emphasize the important qualities a good caregiver should have as well. This will include some of my own behind-the-scenes stories as I explore different models of care and what we can learn from them. Simultaneously, I will highlight the stories of various patients, caregivers, educators, and health professionals who have experienced the system to provide key tips you can use to change your health care experiences.

While this book may initially seem solely for patients who have or are struggling to advocate for themselves in health care settings, it can provide valuable lessons for many roles in the system. Whether you are the caregiver of a patient, a social worker, or an aspiring health professional, this book can provide you with tools to truly understand the mindsets of those who feel silenced by the system and learn about the ways you can enhance the level of communication and engagement you, your loved ones, or your patients receive from those within the system.

Although I cannot control what you do with the information I provide, do me one favor: listen. Listen to the stories of those who have struggled to stand up for themselves while navigating the rocky terrain of the medical system. Listen to the stories of those who have worked for the system and approach their perspectives on how to make it better with an open mind. And if you're extremely dedicated, listen to my perspectives and experiences as a former patient preparing to enter the medical field (although, I'm warning you right now this may come with the occasional funny story, obscure reference, or dad joke). With these diverse perspectives and anecdotes, I hope to empower you to be active in conversations with your health professionals and to get a taste of the care you seek and deserve. While I acknowledge I still have so much to learn about this system myself, I hope this book can be a small step toward fighting for a health care system where curiosity is not seen as a lethal poison. Because, in reality, it's the antidote.

PART I

WHERE WE'VE COME FROM AND WHERE WE'RE HEADED

CHAPTER 1

THE EVOLUTION OF THE DOCTOR-PATIENT RELATIONSHIP

———

If you ask many of my friends what the best place to get baked goods in Miami is, you'll probably get a myriad of answers. Pinecrest Bakery was one of our favorite places near school to get a *cafecito* and some *croquetas*, Fireman Derek's Bake Shop is a go-to spot in Coconut Grove for some delicious pies, and The Salty Donut always has an insane line of customers waiting to devour their artisanal donuts. But weirdly, as I sit in my dorm room in Nashville typing away at this computer, I can't help but think of the delicious double chocolate chip muffins and ham *croquetas* I always ate in the lobby of Nicklaus Children's Hospital while my parents parked the car before my appointments.

While I'm very fortunate to be in good health, I have probably spent more time in health care settings than the average child raised in the United States. Aside from the yearly checkups with my primary care physician, I have annual appointments with a nephrologist because I was born prematurely with a nonfunctional kidney removed at the age of three and an ophthalmologist because of my nearsightedness (I'm pretty much legally blind without corrective lenses—ask anyone who's tried on my glasses for fun). For about eight years, starting in the second grade, I had braces on-and-off and met my orthodontist every three to five months for regular checkups; simultaneously I met with an orthopedist who provided me with a back brace to fix my slight spinal curvature. As I will talk about more later on, I also had surgery during my first year of high school to remove an arteriovenous malformation (AVM) behind my left ear, which required numerous consultations and appointments with a variety of medical professionals, including an otolaryngologist (ear, nose, and throat doctor), neurologist, pulmonologist, and craniofacial surgeon.

Although hospitals and doctors' offices may typically evoke feelings of fear and anxiety, the experience of sitting in the waiting room as I eat my fantastic muffin, watch the *Doc McStuffins* reruns playing on the TV, and wait for someone to loudly proclaim the doctor is ready for their appointment with "Karen Murphy" was oddly relaxing to me. Given that many of my health professionals were long term, we had developed pretty strong relationships and they knew a lot about my personal life and aspirations. As my pediatric nephrologist monitored the condition of my kidney during our yearly appointments, she'd ask me about how school was going and provide me with valuable advice about my aspirations to pursue a health profession. Similarly, when I would visit my orthodontist every few months to monitor and adjust the braces I had worn on-and-off for eight years, he'd always take the time to ask me about my most recent water polo matches and what I expected the season to look like. By taking the time, even if just for a few minutes, to discuss something other than the procedures or diagnostics at hand, Dr. Paredes and Dr. Alquizar really helped me see them as normal human beings, strengthening our rapport and trust in each other. However, the dynamic of my relationship was different with my shorter-term doctors given our shorter time together, which at times made decision-making difficult in moments where it mattered more.

According to Tyler Johnson from the Duke Center for Research on Personalized Health Care, establishing trust and clear communication within the doctor-patient relationship is essential, as "Effective physician-patient communication has been shown to positively influence health outcomes by increasing patient satisfaction, leading to greater patient understanding of health problems and treatments available, contributing to better adherence to treatment plans, and providing support and reassurance to patients."[8] However, factors such as the limited time constraints of appointments, the increased permeation of technology in the health care setting, and general disparities in health communication have made the development of this relationship difficult. In this chapter, I will provide an overview of the evolution of the doctor-patient relationship and the implications this has on being a patient now and in the future.

---

8   Tyler Johnson, "The Importance of Physician-Patient Relationships Communication and Trust in Health Care," Duke Center for Personalized Health Care, last modified March 11, 2019.

A BRIEF HISTORY OF THE DOCTOR-PATIENT RELATIONSHIP

In classical Greek medical theory, disease was hypothesized to originate from the four humors: blood, phlegm, black bile, and yellow bile. These existed in conjunction with four qualities: hot, cold, wet, and dry. Illnesses and health conditions were believed to be heavily influenced by each individual's humoral balance, leading general approaches of treatment and symptom relief to be very personalized in nature.[9]

Until the nineteenth century, people would visit barber surgeons regardless of their illnesses. They would try to alleviate your symptoms but did not attempt to diagnose these errors. One of the first individuals who tried to understand the inner mechanisms that facilitated illness was Leopold Auenbrugger, who developed the technique of percussion to determine the location of the meniscus, after watching his father tap on the sides of wine kegs in their basement. As a physician, he conducted a similar practice that allowed him to determine the relative size of internal organs and the presence of fluid in the lungs. Health professionals embraced a similar approach by placing their ears on the chests of their patients to understand this inner functioning until the development of the stethoscope by René Laennec and other devices such as the ophthalmoscope and the blood pressure cuff.[10]

During a Stanford+Connects micro lecture he gave in Paris, professor and senior associate chair for the Theory and Practice of Medicine, Abraham Verghese, describes the ritualistic nature of the doctor's appointment, which he has explored

---

9   *Stanford Alumni*, "The Doctor-Patient Relationship with Abraham Verghese," October 3, 2013, video, 13:58.

10   Ibid.

with colleagues in anthropology such as Dr. Cari Costanzo Kapur at Stanford. In these moments, patients are immensely vulnerable, as they allow complete strangers to touch their bare bodies to locate an illness. While there may not be a direct cure for their condition, the warmth of the physician's tone and their affirmations of connection and trust validates the patient's personhood, which can provide profound neurobiological effects, a phenomenon he describes as a placebo without a placebo.[11]

The development of such technologies and techniques creates a shift in the power dynamic between physicians and patients. During times when patients primarily believed in nonmedical sources of illnesses, the role of physicians was not admired to the same degree it is now, with patients having the power to interpret their illness and choosing whether or not to employ a physician. However, the "pendulum of power" shifted with the rise of hospital medicine and increasingly secular beliefs with regards to medicine. As a result, medicine became increasingly depersonalized, as the focus shifted from the patients' narratives to data rendered from medical technologies.[12]

"This notion was explored by writer Hervé Guibert in his description of the famous French philosopher Michel Foucault's experience of being treated in hospital for HIV/AIDS in early 1990s France: Foucault 'spent a morning in the hospital having tests done, and told me he'd forgotten how completely the body loses all identity once it's delivered into

---

11   Ibid.

12   Natalie Harrison, "Regressing or progressing: what next for the doctor-patient relationship?," *The Lancet* 6, 3(2018):178-180.

medical hands, becoming just a package of helpless flesh, trundled around here and there, hardly even a number on a slip of paper.' Elsner notes that this example is paradigmatic of the doctor-patient relationship in the latter half of the 20th century, capturing the dehumanizing effects of Foucault's concept of the 'medical gaze'—the medical separation of the patient's body from the patient's person and identity."[13]

While the implementation of a myriad of medical technologies has contributed to the relative weakening of the doctor-patient relationship, many physicians have also found current policies and protocols to be similarly restrictive and frustrating. Many doctors are required to fulfill certain quotas that promote examining the maximum number of patients possible, but their visits are often only limited to about fifteen to twenty minutes of conversation. This makes it much more difficult to establish a strong rapport with their patients, which is especially crucial when rapid decisions need to be made.

During an interview with Dr. Gary Siegel, a specialist in anesthesiology and pain medicine, we had an interesting conversation regarding a hospital policy that concerns patients who do not speak English. To create opportunities for conversation with these patients, the hospital requires its employees to use an interpreter service on a tablet. While we agreed this policy was important and has many beneficial elements, including providing patients with the comfort of care in their native tongue and limiting any liabilities caused by miscommunication, Dr. Siegel simultaneously expressed some concerns surrounding various restrictions that have

---

13   Ibid.

also arisen as a result. Despite being a fluent Spanish speaker, he is not allowed to converse with the patients in their preferred language without the interpreter service present, which has malfunctioned numerous times during appointments if there are connectivity issues. In certain ways, the policy creates a barrier for physicians who are actually capable of facilitating more organic conversations with their patients, leaving Dr. Siegel and others feeling rather disconnected from these patients.

"My enjoyment in what I do is establishing relationships with human beings. You know, it's not sticking needles in people or pushing meds in an IV or looking at a monitor to correct vital signs. It's the human-to-human part. And so when I have to deal with technical issues with the interpreter service, it's horrible. It takes the human-to-human part away, especially as far as different cultural issues and sensitivities to that."

Although such policies may be immensely beneficial for physicians who do not speak the languages of those whom they serve, it is important to interrogate these policies' influences on the doctor-patient relationship by holistically considering all the consequences that result from their implementation. As the medical profession has become increasingly bureaucratic and technological in nature, both physicians and patients alike have become increasingly frustrated and appear to demonstrate a mutual desire to return genuine human connection to the forefront of health care. For this reason, it is essential to consider the doctor-patient relationship when crafting policy to facilitate the best opportunities for both parties and develop a sense of rapport and trust as they navigate the terrain ahead together.

TRANSITIONS TO TELEHEALTH AND THE WAKE OF COVID-19

Given the unique circumstances surrounding the COVID-19 pandemic, both emotional and physical distance have been further exacerbated by social distancing protocols. Although hospitals still function and run, the number of visitors has been substantially limited and many physicians have transitioned consultations and appointments by using telehealth techniques. This has provided a unique challenge for physicians to go the distance during social distancing, as they must conduct thorough and comprehensive assessments of their patients without the ability to directly use many medical technologies to provide accurate diagnoses. Additionally, many nonverbal cues that often convey empathy and compassion are limited by the constraints of their cameras during telehealth appointments and even in person given the necessary use of masks. However, while these circumstances have increased the physical distance between patients and doctors alike, they have simultaneously created new environments in which patients may be more comfortable conversing with their health professionals, especially given they can meet with them virtually, in the comfort of their own home.

Because of the general hysteria surrounding the pandemic and the dramatic lifestyle changes associated with maintaining protocols to prevent the spread of the virus, mental health has also become a key health concern that cannot be swept under the rug. With many people undergoing financial difficulties and others being forced to return to hostile home environments where they experience abuse or discrimination based on their sexual orientations, among many other factors, developing genuine emotional connections, especially with health professionals, is of immediate and grand importance to maintaining our collective well-being of individuals during the pandemic.

"At this moment, all we have to give to our patients is ourselves. The fact that the doctor is risking his own health to be there to take the burden of suffering away is the art in its purest form. The compassion to see this patient as a unique person is truly an art that can never be taught in school or learned from a textbook. Knowing they are not alone and with someone who is truly there for them is all that can be done at this moment."

— DR. MICHAEL C. LUCIANO[14]

Now that you have a general understanding of the dynamic nature of the doctor-patient relationship, both throughout history and within the modern climate, we will move on to actionable ways in which patients, their loved ones, and physicians alike can mitigate these barriers to creating genuine emotional connections with each other in health care settings.

---

14   Michael C. Luciano, "The Art of the Doctor-Patient Relationship in the COVID-19 Era," MEDPAGE TODAY, last modified April 23, 2020.

CHAPTER 2

UNMASKING AUTONOMY: WHY WE CRAVE CONTROL

Although at times mundane, the mandatory quarantine period my friends and I jokingly called our "Coronacation" (that began, of course, with "the year of March") provided a unique opportunity to discover many new things. One thing I learned very quickly after my favorite childhood television show, *Avatar: The Last Airbender*, hit Netflix in May was it is somehow even better upon rewatching. The movie adaptation, however, was just as, if not more disappointing as it was the first time, and I just got that from accidentally watching the trailer (seriously, if you did not cringe every other minute of this movie, I recommend you seek some form of counseling and I stand by that opinion). In other news, I also discovered my new favorite bakery item: cronuts.

Not only is the word "cronut" fun to say, but these delicious pastries best served warm combine both the amazing sugary taste of a good donut and the flaky, light texture of a croissant, leading to a symphony of delicious flavors delighting your taste buds. Upon having these on a few occasions during the summer, I was excited to find the best cronut spots when I returned to Nashville to begin my sophomore year at Vanderbilt.

After unpacking all of my boxes, showing my mother some of my favorite restaurants around campus, as well the Parthenon where the first *Percy Jackson* movie was filmed, we decided to go to a local bakery to pick up some cronuts before she had to leave for the airport. I ordered a Lyft on my phone and we hopped into a gray Honda Civic, excited to satiate our craving. Our driver, a man named Arthur, was very kind and asked me some questions about how I was enjoying Vanderbilt and what I looked forward to in the coming year. However, what came out of his mouth next was a shock to both me and my mother.

"So what are your thoughts on this whole pandemic thing? Because, frankly, I think wearing masks is a bunch of bullshit."

My mom and I looked at each other confused and somewhat uncomfortable as Arthur spoke lengthily on how he believed masks were just a means of us showing obedience to our government and how wearing them went against his values. A devout Christian, he told us God made people to be loving and affectionate and masks were preventing people from doing that. Arthur proclaimed if mask regulations were not lifted by January 1, 2021, he would throw his in the fire and go hug his loved ones.

Knowing I was a premedical student, he asked me if I thought masks were really doing anything for our health. At this point, I had a lot of strong opinions against what he said that I was ready to voice. But I could tell he didn't want to know what I had to say and instead decided to respond by simply saying, "Yes, I really do believe they are beneficial." We bade him a good day and quickly left the car, both a little alarmed by Arthur's sentiments, but still unwavering in our firm belief masks were a key component in addressing the COVID-19 pandemic.

Studies have indicated wearing a mask, whether it be a cloth, surgical, or N95 respiratory mask, has been able to reduce the risk of infection by respiratory virus emitted in droplets or aerosols.[15] One study even found saying a simple phrase generated droplets ranging from twenty to five hundred micrometers, but simply covering the speaker's mouth with a slightly damp washcloth curbed the number of forward-moving droplets.[16] While it is most beneficial for those actually infected with the virus to wear them to prevent infection of others, the asymptomatic nature of many cases has led even those who have not been feeling ill to adopt the practice. Many people, including some of my close friends, have also used masks to complement their personal fashion choices by sewing their own masks or purchasing ones with their favorite designs and logos. Yet, despite the extensive

---

15   Nina Bai, "Still Confused About Masks? Here's the Science Behind How Face Masks Prevent Coronavirus," UCSF, last modified July 11, 2020.

16   Philip Anfinrund et al., "Visualizing Speech-Generated Oral Fluid Droplets with Laser Light Scattering," *The New England Journal of Medicine* 382, 21(2020):2061-2063.

research and science that support this practice, there are still many individuals who refuse to wear masks.

Those who are colloquially referred to as "anti-maskers" cite many reasons as to why they refuse to cover their faces in public spaces. Various people, like Arthur, have told me they believe wearing masks is a sign of government compliance and infringes on their civil liberties. Others have claimed it is a sign of fear and weakness; they believe opposing the protocols is a sign of strength and immunity to the virus. And some just don't understand how the act of wearing a mask is helping anything—aren't people still dying anyway?

As someone who is very pro-mask, the justifications provided by those who choose not to wear masks initially both confused and frustrated me. Every time I saw someone without their mask or wearing it incorrectly, many thoughts would race through my mind. *How can these people be so insensitive and selfish? Why is wearing a singular piece of cloth so difficult for some people to do? Does our society really have such little regard for human life?*

I will admit many of my thoughts, along with those aforementioned, were quite aggressive given my very strong alignment with science and public health. While I am not the biggest fan of wearing a mask for prolonged periods of time, I saw it as my duty to protect myself from exposure, and consequently, my loved ones and their loved ones as well. While I honestly rolled my eyes after reading many of the excuses individuals had for not wearing masks, I was particularly struck by one quote from a *Huffington Post* article I read on my phone one day as I walked toward my dad's store:

"So much is uncertain right now. It makes me feel in control to choose to go out without a mask."[17]

Interestingly, this statement did not provoke any sort of anger or hostility as I read it. Rather, my frustration was swiftly redirected into empathy and curiosity and I decided to read on. Joseph K. Trunzo, a psychology professor and department chair of Bryant University in Smithfield, Rhode Island, explained in a time period so turbulent and uncertain as the one we live in, we seek a need for control to cope with our fear.

"When faced with uncertain situations over which we have no control, we tend to exercise it wherever we can, so we feel safe...Some will feel safer exercising their control over not wearing a mask, while others will feel safer exercising their control to wear one."[18]

When confronted with opinions that are different from our own, it is very easy to put up a wall and completely disregard the opposing side. As someone who has engaged in numerous debates with close family and friends, ranging from arguments regarding views on political policies, surrounding accessibility to medical care, and to whether Ross and Rachel were on a break or not in *Friends* (they were definitely on a break, of course, although I do think Ross acted a bit rashly). However, this time I really tried to wrap my head around this opposing point of view.

---

17   Brittany Wong, "The Psychology Behind Why Some People Refuse To Wear Face Masks," *HuffPost*, July 01, 2020.

18   Ibid.

In many ways, those who are pro-mask and anti-mask essentially form two opposing sides of the same coin. Everyone's situation is definitely unique, but we live with the same fear and uncertainty regarding what comes next. *How much longer will we have to adhere to social distancing protocols? When will scientists release a viable vaccine? Will things ever go back to normal?*

Having a fear of the unknown is very common and given the current political, environmental, and social climates, people find it even more essential to have a sense of control and security in their lives. For some, the desire for control is satiated by following the protocols recommended by the Centers for Disease Control and Prevention (CDC), as they find empowerment in holding themselves accountable for their safety through concrete action. For others, this overwhelming confusion and uncertainty make it difficult for them to know who to trust. They find control by doing what they feel is inherently correct, which, for some, means not wearing a mask. And of course, there are just some people who don't like being told what to do, and their sense of confidence and independence provides them with the security and means to navigate uncertain scenarios.

By writing about this topic, I am by no means trying to rationalize the decision to not wear a mask nor am I encouraging others to follow suit. I chose to mention this to elucidate the impact of having perceived control in the face of uncertainty and how it can motivate our behavior. To further this point, I will use this chapter to explore how taking ownership of our decisions can substantially influence our subsequent behaviors related to such choices.

THE CHOICES FROM WITHIN

The idea of taking ownership of one's decisions seems deceptively simple.

Sure, you chose to eat a salad for lunch today instead of the delicious fried chicken in the dining hall, but was it because you were craving a crisp piece of romaine lettuce or was it the looming, condescending eyes of the server who could tell the jeans you were wearing were a little too snug? At the end of the day, you may feel good about yourself for choosing a healthier meal, but if you are anything like myself, it won't be long before you're in your kitchen that same night eating spoons of Nutella straight from the jar without fear of judgment since everyone else in the house is asleep. Although the influence of others can help steer you to make certain choices, it is only when you take ownership of the decisions you make they really become yours.

While many of the decisions we make on a daily basis are surrounded by external factors for motivation, many investigations have found our behaviors are most impactful when the drive comes from within. One iconic study examining this phenomenon was conducted in 1962 by Dr. Sam Glucksberg, a psychology professor at Princeton University, during which he presented students with the "Candle Problem." Each student was provided with a thumbtack box with about fifty thumbtacks in it, some matches, and a wax candle, the latter of which they were asked to mount on the wall given the materials provided. If students tried to melt a side of the candle and adhere it to the wall, its weight made it fall, and nailing the candle directly to the wall was unsuccessful as the candle's flaky structure would make it crumble.

The answer to this problem was simply emptying the thumb-tack box, tacking it to the wall, and mounting the candle on top of the box by slightly melting the base of the candle. The initial purpose of presenting individuals with the candle problem was to examine if they could overcome functional fixedness, or the idea certain objects only have a singular intended purpose. When the box was presented to students without the tacks in it, they finished the task much quicker, no longer seeing the box as solely a container for the tacks.

Glucksberg's twist, however, was introducing a financial incentive to the picture. While he tasked half of the participants with solely solving the problem, he told the other group they could win five dollars or twenty dollars based on how quickly they solved it in comparison to their peers, a pretty great prize for a college student in the 1960s (as a current college student myself in 2021, it's still a pretty nice reward for a few minutes of work). Not surprisingly, when the box was presented without the tacks, the cash incentive led many students to finish the task very quickly as compared to their peers who were not offered anything. However, when both groups were presented with the box filled with thumbtacks, in which their creativity was challenged, the money prize actually increased the time students took to finish the task by about three and a half minutes.[19]

As stated perfectly in an article from the nonprofit online magazine *Behavioral Scientist,* "Paradoxically, stronger motivation decreases insightfulness," with motivation in this case

---

19   John Kounios and Mark Beeman, "How Incentives Hinder Innovation," *Behavioral Scientist,* September 03, 2015.

referring to extrinsic factors such as financial incentives and deadlines.[20] Although relatively analytical and mundane tasks can be done quicker under similar external pressures, the same cannot be said for activities and decisions that require ingenuity or lack a cookie cutter answer.

Let's return to salads. Say you are tasked with preparing a Caesar salad in under ten minutes for one hundred dollars. That should be relatively easy, right? Basically, you could just add some leafy lettuce, cheese, and croutons and toss them all quickly in some store-brand Caesar dressing. If you're feeling a little risqué, maybe add some olive oil and avocado to mix things up.

Now what if you were asked to make the perfect Caesar salad for one thousand dollars you know will be judged among about one hundred others? The stakes have gotten much higher. At this point, you consider adding chicken to provide some extra protein. Maybe you want to make the Caesar dressing from scratch. You're suddenly confident your cooking skills are superior to whoever made the dressing you grabbed from the middle shelf at Target because it was embarrassing to jump and reach for the slightly cheaper bottle on the top shelf (this may or may not be based on a true story). You also decide to get some black pepper and garlic to make your otherwise bland salad nice and spicy.

But let's not forget the twist. Like everyone else, you only have ten minutes. Suddenly, you don't have time to make dressing from scratch and can't take the time to massage

---

20   Ibid.

each individual leaf so the dressing to oil ratio is perfect. Disheartened, you turn in your subpar attempt to recreate the perfect salad that has now become a bitter memory in your head.

Now, as sad as you may feel right now having lost the chance of hypothetically winning one thousand dollars for your hypothetical salad, I want you to go back and remember what it felt like for those brief moments where the deadline and the money were out of the picture. Think about the amazing tastes you expected to enjoy as you chewed each tasty bite. Recognize and appreciate the saliva that has now collected in your mouth that may hypothetically be dripping on your computer keyboard as you type this story for your book. While you may taste some amazing salads in your life, none of them will ever come close to this one.

The best decisions in your life are not ones made for money, on a deadline, or to please others. Like salads, the best choices you will ever make, the ones you can truly call yours, are the ones that come from within.

WHY TOO MUCH CHOICE IS A RECIPE FOR DISASTER AND THE PRESCRIPTION FOR SUCCESS

So you might be asking yourself, why is this man talking about candles and condiments in a book about making health care decisions?

As I attempted to illustrate through my salad scenario (don't worry, for both of our sakes salads will not be mentioned for the remainder of this book), a barrier that often daunts those who seek autonomy at times is, well, too much freedom.

As American psychologist Barry Schwartz explores in his book *The Paradox of Choice* (2004), the presence of too many options can sometimes induce paralysis, rather than liberation. We are left pondering a myriad of different pathways that could result from a singular decision, from small choices like picking a city to pursue your career, to monumental ones like deciding which ice cream flavor to get when you finally reach the front of the line (I joke, of course, but frankly a poor choice in ice cream can really ruin your whole day).

Now, take a second and substitute the ice cream flavors with different cancer treatment approaches. The decision between chocolate, vanilla, and strawberry now becomes one of elective surgery, chemotherapy, and medication. For patients presented with potentially life-threatening diagnoses, the clock becomes much more important, with swift responses becoming key in preventing illnesses from drastically escalating, and the whirlwind of emotions making it even more difficult to make an informed, clear decision about one's health.

Health professionals can serve as immensely valuable assets in helping their patients navigate these difficult scenarios. One method providers can use is called shared decision making. This technique empowers patients to become more engaged in decision making, while also reminding them they are not alone: their health professionals will be there to support them every step of the way by providing insight based on their knowledge of the field and teaching skills to help them manage their conditions.

According to Lane Stiles, former Director of Patient Education at Vanderbilt University Medical Center, one of the most important elements of this method is it reminds patients they have a role in their health and well-being and they matter. A shocking statistic he shared with me during an interview was one out of every three prescriptions for new diagnoses for hypertension and diabetes are never filled, much less used the way they should be used. A big reason for that is patients feel like they don't own their decisions.

"Somebody made the decision for them and told them to get this prescription but they don't own it. They don't feel it yet. They haven't said 'I need to do this.'"

But when balance between autonomy and guidance is achieved by health professionals *and* patients, it creates a much better opportunity for patients to follow through and hold themselves accountable for their care. For example, let's look at the story of Julie, a member of the Diabetes Advisory Council for Mayo Clinic in Minnesota. In her story, she shares that while she had been seeing a primary care physician for the last eight years, she had not really been taking her care as seriously as she does now.

"I wasn't having any symptoms. It really wasn't showing up so I kind of ignored it."[21]

However, she was referred to an endocrinologist who embraced the mentality of shared decision making and really made a difference in her care.

---

21 *Mayo Clinic,* "Patient Experience with Shared Decision Making at Mayo Clinic," December 28, 2010, video, 3:37.

"It wasn't somebody saying here's what you should do; it was a difference of saying here's all the options (and there's lots of options) and now let's talk about what makes sense for you."[22]

With her health professional's knowledge of her condition and recognition she as the patient knew what would best fit her lifestyle, Julie was able to find the best plan for herself to manage her diabetes. While it took her a bit more time at first to understand things and develop rapport with her doctor, she now feels much more empowered to research, talk with others who share the same chronic condition, and to ask the questions she needs answers for to leave her appointments without any regrets.

"What I found is that actually being part of that decision-making process I have held closer to the treatment, that I should stay with, not to say I do everything perfect, but I am a well-controlled type two diabetic now and I can tell I'm living healthier and I know that will make a difference for me in the long run."[23]

Julie's story, among the others presented in this chapter, reminds us the simple act of making a choice, regardless of how big or small, inherently empowers us. When we actually make decisions on our own terms, whether it be as small as choosing a salad dressing or as large as determining one's treatment plan, we are much more likely to take ownership of our actions and put forth our best effort, creating more chances for positive outcomes or at least valuable learning

---

22   Ibid.
23   Ibid.

opportunities. With the right balance of intrinsic motivation and extrinsic support, especially in health-related situations, we are equipped with a recipe for success to exercise our autonomy and make informed decisions that are in our best interests.

CHAPTER 3

THE IMPORTANCE OF HEALTH EDUCATION

———

As reigning regional champions in the health education category of Future Health Professionals' (HOSA) annual competition, my partner Julio and I were excited to compete again during our junior year of high school, in hopes of regaining our title. Given that numerous schedule conflicts and other commitments prevented us from competing at the state level the year prior, we had our eyes on qualifying for states again and even potentially nationals.

During our sophomore year of high school, we decided to curate a health education lesson for fifth grade students focused on nutrition and dental hygiene. While the lesson was a popular choice for many health education initiatives, both in our competition and in general, we were praised by our judges for incorporating creative activities that had tangible applications to real life skills, such as teaching our students how to interpret the categories on food labels and using them to evaluate common snacks they usually ate.

Our primary activity, however, had students try different methods of teeth brushing by coating hard-boiled eggs with Glo Germ, a powder product that fluoresces under UV light, commonly used to teach hand washing. By experimenting with brushing with swirls, including water, or holding the toothbrush at different angles, the scholars were able to directly witness the importance of thoroughly brushing every day and were able to better appreciate learning some fundamentals of dental hygiene, rather than hearing us lecture off our slides.

As juniors, we were particularly inspired by a screening of the movie *Contagion* in our medical interventions class, deciding to curate a lesson on the different methods of disease transmission and preventative measures. We again tried to challenge ourselves to incorporate creative and fun approaches to breaking down this topic in our lesson plan, including playing with bubble guns to represent the transmission of airborne diseases and using an activity from the CDC that requires students to determine the source of an outbreak at a carnival, where a virus rapidly infects people by turning them into flesh-eating zombies.

Given our previous success and the addition of another friend of ours to the team, we went in relatively confident we would be able to place again and hopefully secure the gold medal. After leaving our presentation, which we felt relatively good about, we ran into another group who enthusiastically asked us about our topic. As we told them about our ideas and asked about theirs, one of the members solely told us, "FGM, look it up," right before they quickly entered the classroom to present their lesson plan to the judges.

Confused, my partners and I quickly looked up FGM on our phones and realized they were presenting a health education lesson on female genital mutilation, the cutting or removal of portions of or the entire external female genitalia. All of us looked at each other in confusion and wondered how this was relevant to a health education lesson. However, upon doing some further research, we realized this practice was highly controversial and illegal in the United States, with FGM being most prevalent in refugee populations, especially in East Africa. This practice has been shaped by numerous cultural and social norms of the areas where it is enforced, and according to the CDC, can lead to numerous averse health consequences, including increasing the risk of death for the mother and her infant(s) during subsequent pregnancy, post-traumatic stress disorder (PTSD), urinary tract infections (UTIs), and many more, aside from the potential negative consequences this may also have on the woman's sexual health.[24]

It was in that moment I was truly able to comprehend the intersectional nature of health. While we are taught so much about basic anatomy and biology, there are so many sociocultural dimensions that influence the health and well-being of individuals around the world and perpetuate the disparities unfortunately plaguing many marginalized populations. Reflecting on that experience, I am disappointed I reacted with such shock and confusion upon seeing a topic like female genital mutilation in a health curriculum. Discussions surrounding topics such as cultural practices and social structures along with the disproportionate impact of numerous

---

24   Center for Disease Control and Prevention, "Female Genital Cutting," accessed October 29, 2020.

illnesses and conditions on communities based on race, sexual orientation, and socioeconomic status should be normalized before students reach the college level, especially considering those who may not be interested in pursuing a health-related career may never hear about them at all. Through this chapter, I will provide a brief commentary on the nature of health education in the United States, including testimonies from my own teachers, to evaluate the current curricula in place and suggest important future areas of exploration that should be implemented and normalized in such programs.

A BRIEF HISTORY OF HEALTH EDUCATION
IN THE UNITED STATES OF AMERICA

Prior to the mid-nineteenth century, initiatives promoting health education in school settings were relatively sparse and uncommon. While Benjamin Franklin supported implementing physical exercise as a primary subject in schools during his time, it was not until 1850 the modern school health era began, during which the Sanitary Commission of Massachusetts, led by Lemuel Shattuck, released an important report that still remains a classic in the field of public health.[25] By releasing this report, public education settings and school programs became a target for health promotion and disease prevention, with key facets of their mission embodied in the following excerpt:

"Every child should be taught early in life, that, to preserve his own life and his own health and the lives and health of others, is one of the most important and constantly abiding duties.

---

25   Diane Allensworth, eds., Elaine Lawson, eds., Lois Nicholson, eds., and James Wyche, eds., *Schools and Health: Our Nation's Investment* (Washington DC: National Academies Press, 1997).

By obeying certain laws or performing certain acts, his life and health may be preserved; by disobedience, or performing certain other acts, they will both be destroyed. By knowing and avoiding the causes of disease, disease itself will be avoided, and he may enjoy health and live; by ignorance of these causes and exposure to them, he may contract disease, ruin his health, and die. Everything connected with wealth, happiness and long life depends upon health; and even the great duties of morals and religion are performed more acceptably in a healthy than a sickly condition."[26]

The temperance movement simultaneously influenced health curricula during the mid-nineteenth and early-twentieth centuries, which stressed the importance of educating children on how substances such as alcohol, narcotics, and tobacco impacted human body systems. This, coupled with various public health epidemics, led to further implementation of initiatives to promote good hygiene and physical training to maintain a strong immune system. Efforts were also focused on improving accessibility to health-related services within school settings.

In 1928, the *Sixth Yearbook* of the Department of Superintendence of the National Education Association published content guidelines for health education, emphasizing the following:

"

- Mental hygiene must be emphasized and protected.

---

26   Ibid.

- The establishment of health habits depends upon the pupil's understanding something of the function of his own body.
- A discussion of the causes of disease merits a place in the secondary school program.
- A thorough study of nutrition should be placed in the upper grades.
- Posture should be emphasized.
- The hygiene of the home should be taught.
- Sex hygiene cannot be overlooked.

27"

In addition to these key areas, health education in the form of safety became increasingly implemented into curricula, with topics such as fire prevention, traffic safety, and bicycle safety becoming integrated into classrooms. During the mid-twentieth century, adolescent health issues entered the foreground, with schools beginning to tackle mental, social, and emotional health issues as well as criminal behavior, substance abuse, and difficulties in adapting to school environments.[28]

However, while such efforts existed and continue to ground health education programs, the focus has shifted more toward skill-based health education, providing students with specific behaviors and mindsets that will allow them to maintain and enhance their well-being outside of the classroom setting. This shift is visible when comparing the guidelines

---

27   Ibid.
28   Ibid.

presented earlier to the following *Characteristics of Effective Health Education Curricula* published by the CDC in 2015, which include:

"

- Provides functional health knowledge that is basic, accurate and directly contributes to health-promoting decisions and behaviors;
- Builds personal competence, social competence, and self-efficacy by addressing skills;
- Provides opportunities to reinforce skills and positive health behaviors

29"

Rather than solely emphasizing topics that should be discussed, effective curricula are now expected to prepare students to act upon the information they learn through both in-class activities and in daily life choices. By doing so, curricula give students the opportunity to practice positive health behaviors within a classroom setting and allow the instructor to help students refine such skills and effectively integrate them into their daily lifestyles, until they almost become muscle memory.

However, this is not to say current curricula are by any means perfect or lack room for growth and refinement. Although health education initiatives have continued to evolve and improve, multiple barriers have compromised the quality of and attention directed toward it. As mandates such as the

---

29   Ibid.

federal No Child Left Behind Act and Every Student Succeeds Act have increased the attention directed toward English Language Arts (ELA) and math education, subjects considered outside of the "core," such as the arts and even health education, have been compromised. Data from the School Health Policies and Practices Study (SHPPS) shows, "instruction in health topics such as alcohol and other drug use prevention, HIV prevention, infectious disease prevention, and tobacco use prevention has decreased" since 2000.[30]

Additionally, numerous topics have been increasingly politicized and subject to debate. Sexual health education varies across the nation, with approaches ranging from focuses on prevention, to biological understanding, to abstinence, leaving some students feeling relatively unequipped to approach these situations within their daily lives. While conversations surrounding mental health have improved, a level of stigma remains surrounding conditions of this nature that makes it difficult to discuss these issues in complete transparency. In addition to these two important concerns, there is also a need to address the importance of intersectionality in health education, with important areas such as socioeconomic status, sexual orientation, and racial and ethnic disparities not often at the forefront of the conversation.

In addition to the exploration of such issues, health education itself is not always a requirement at each school. For example, at my high school, I was granted an exemption from taking health class because I participated in the

---

30   Donna M. Videto and Joseph A. Drake. "Promoting Health Literacy Through Defining and Measuring Quality School Health Education." *Health Promotion Practice* 20, 6(2019):824-833.

International Baccalaureate program, which does not typically require health education courses. Although I took advantage of this policy and used my newfound schedule's flexibility to take more classes in biomedical and natural science, I am not a strong proponent of it. During a conversation with the health education teacher at my high school, Mrs. Suzanne Landsom, she discussed a similar frustration with both the short duration allotted to her health class (one semester) and the ability for students to bypass the requirement.

"I am not a fan of a student being exempt from health especially with the current state of adolescents with regard to increases in depression, suicide, obesity, sexually transmitted diseases, alcohol, and drug use. The students really need to understand that my class helps them better understand the pressures of being a teenager or young adult. My students are learning about things that they will take with them throughout their entire lives regardless of their career choices."

While I took numerous biology, anatomy, and biomedical science classes that covered many health-related topics, I definitely would have benefitted from the more specific and targeted health education class I did not take. This need is probably even stronger for students who similarly did not take health class, but also lack an affinity or interest in health-related courses, opting to focus their efforts on the humanities or social sciences, for example. Creating access to curricula focused on transforming students into active participants in their own health care and the care of others is invaluable and facilitates the development of important skills they can carry into adulthood.

FUTURE DIRECTIONS TO EXPLORE
IN HEALTH EDUCATION CURRICULA

One of my favorite classes I took in high school was "Principles of Biomedical Science" during ninth grade, in which we had to follow the mysterious death of a fictional woman named Anna Garcia. At the beginning of the course, we dipped our toes into some introductory procedures involved in forensic science, such as fingerprint matching, witness and suspect accounts, and one of my personal favorites, blood spatter analysis. However, as we received more information about Anna and her medical history, we began exploring different testing procedures, medical conditions, and human body systems.

While we completed many interesting projects throughout the year, one that particularly stuck with me that my teacher, Mrs. Yoly McCarthy, continues to assign her students every year, is the creation of a recipe that would be a delicious and nutritious food option for someone who has diabetes. Once we all developed our recipe and brought samples for the entire class, she compiled them into a diabetes-friendly class cookbook. While we learned a lot about the hormonal pathways and underlying biology behind the condition, this project provided a direct application to the lifestyle of an individual with Type one or Type two diabetes, challenging us to look beyond the content and engage in creative problem solving, as we navigated the everyday choices an individual living with either condition had to make regarding their diet. Although our products were truthfully not the most delicious (Mrs. McCarthy told me later she especially dreads having to try another student's painful attempt at avocado brownies), many of my classmates and I left appreciative of the opportunity we had, to take what we learned in the classroom and directly apply it to a real-life situation.

As I caught up with Mrs. McCarthy this past summer and reminisced about my time in her class, she told me more about why she incorporates so many interactive activities into her class curriculum.

"In many cases, the kids think that they're not qualified enough, not smart enough, not in a good enough position to have ownership of knowledge that they know. They say that it should be the teacher telling me what to do and all I'm doing is answering questions from the book. You know, the textbook tells me what to do and the teacher manages me. That's wrong. That's not education. That's babysitting. True education comes when the student becomes the teacher per se and is able to do something with the information—apply it not just to a new situation, but is able to make it something new. Make it understandable for somebody else. And that right there is the biggest factor."

When I brought up this conversation with my developmental editor, she was reminded of the idea of home economics classes. While we both have many qualms with the home economics class model as a whole, which are unsurprisingly shared by many and have led to their decrease in prevalence in recent years, there is something positive to be said about incorporating programs in education settings that provide students with functional knowledge and skills they can directly apply to real-life situations. Although health education models have provided students with valuable information about regulating their diets and conducting exercise, there are so many other important health-related skills that could be taught earlier, with some particularly important examples provided below.

UNDERSTANDING HEALTH INSURANCE.

Other than the times when I have sought out information for myself or had small discussions about accessibility in some of my classes, I have never really learned how health insurance works or what it covers. Oftentimes, people are fine with solely knowing about whether they have insurance or not, but concerns surrounding coverage only begin to arise when someone close to them are in a compromising situation, at which point it may be too late. Given the extensive nature of the topic and my own faults in understanding, I have provided some resources at the end of this chapter that may be useful for those of you who would like to understand the basics of health insurance.

COMMUNICATING WITH HEALTH PROFESSIONALS.

It would be incredible to have modules or lessons embedded within health education curricula that directly address the process of conversing with a health professional. While children often learn how to speak to their doctors from observing their family members, providing them with even the most basic skills and foundations to advocate for themselves would be immensely useful if or once they become the primary communicator with their health professionals. According to numerous accounts I have heard from friends and family alike, they became involved and inquisitive during conversations with their health professionals only after they had left an appointment either confused about what they had heard or disappointed in themselves for not asking a question they needed an answer to. It should not have to take a negative experience for an individual to learn how to speak to their medical professional; while these situations may arise at times due to the fault of the health care provider, communication is a two-way street that still requires patients to take initiative, especially when they feel they aren't being heard.

IMPROVING STATISTICAL ILLITERACY.
While statistics have increasingly become implemented in both premedical and mathematical education, both patients and physicians alike have been shown to struggle at times with numeracy, a tactic often manipulated by pharmaceutical commercials. An article written by Gerd Gigerenzer et al. titled "Helping Doctors and Patients Make Sense of Health Statistics" highlights our collective statistical illiteracy as a society, or "the widespread inability to understand the meaning of numbers."[31] A particularly alarming instance they mentioned to elucidate this issue occurred in 1995, when the UK Committee on Safety of Medications issued a warning regarding the potential of oral contraceptive pills to increase the risk of potentially life-threatening blood clots. While the absolute risk in reality changed from one in every seven thousand women having a thrombosis to two in every seven thousand women, this was advertised in terms of relative risk, leading people to believe the risk had increased by two-fold, or 100 percent. This provoked substantial anxiety nationwide as women abandoned the pill, which increased both unwanted pregnancies and abortions (an estimated thirteen thousand additional abortions were performed in England and Wales

---

31   Gerd Gigerenzer et al., "Helping Doctors and Patients Make Sense of Health Statistics," *Psychological Science in the Public Interest* 8, 2(2007):53-96.

during the following year).[32] By increasing education surrounding the statistics of risk and odds, especially related to health, many harmful misconceptions could be avoided and the duality of health care delivery and experiences could be dramatically enhanced for both patients and physicians alike.

As you may have guessed, my group and I placed second in the Health Education category and qualified for states, which we were again unable to attend due to some logistical conflicts. I would like to think the group presenting on FGM had won, but unfortunately, I had never gotten their names and could not recognize their faces at the awards ceremony that took place about a month after the competition. Nonetheless, I am immensely grateful for having run into them and competed alongside individuals who were already identifying and educating fellow students on health issues I am now so passionate about. As I continue my academic endeavors, I hope to continue learning more about intersectional public health issues and educating others about their prevalence so we can collectively engage in efforts to improve the quality of life and health for individuals worldwide.

RESOURCES FOR UNDERSTANDING HEALTH INSURANCE

While I still have much to learn, here are some resources I found helpful in beginning to understand and navigate the world of health insurance.

- **"The Complete Guide to Health Insurance" by Jennifer McCarthy (Free).** This article on The Simple Dollar website provides a comprehensive yet understandable

---

32   Ibid.

overview of what health insurance is and how it works. I would definitely recommend reading it if you are interested![33]

- **"Financial Advocacy in Rare: Navigating the US Health System for Young Adults" by Sophie Pieri (Free).** This toolkit created by Global Genes consists of personal anecdotes, tips, resources, and suggestions to best advocate for yourself and your loved ones as you navigate health insurance. Although their resources are primarily directed to individuals and their loved ones in the rare disease community, there is still a lot that can be learned from the resources they provide.[34]

- https://globalgenes.happyfox.com/kb/article/26-navigating-health-insurance/

- **"Navigating Health Insurance" by Harvard Health Publishing ($18).** This paid guide provides targeted descriptions and resources that will help you understand your hospital bills, navigate your charges, and compare health plans.[35]

---

33 Jennifer McCarthy, "The Complete Guide to Health Insurance," The Simple Dollar, last modified August 28, 2020.

34 Sophie Pieri, "Navigating Health Insurance," Global Genes, last modified February 09, 2021.

35 Harvard Health, "Navigating Health Insurance," accessed December 26, 2020.

PART II

THE CURIOUS PATIENT

CHAPTER 4

(EMOTIONAL) ROLLERCOASTERS: THE DROPS, LOOPS, AND TURNS

———

Raised in Miami, Florida for the majority of my childhood, I had many opportunities to visit the amazing amusement parks in Orlando, given it took just a few hours to drive there. On a few occasions in elementary school, my parents gave me the options of either organizing a big birthday with my classmates or driving up to Walt Disney World for the weekend with my grandfather. Enamored by the incredible atmosphere of amusement parks, I picked the latter whenever given the opportunity and still cherish the fond memories of sharing a turkey leg with my dad, as my mom often unsuccessfully tried to navigate us to the nearest ride.

However, despite the many trips I took to these parks both as a child and later as an adolescent to compete in water polo tournaments, I was always too scared to ride the large rollercoasters. Looking back on it, I honestly had no idea what was really stopping me. Maybe it was the intimidating nature of the rides' tall structures (but given my short height even now, most things just seem tall), or perhaps it came from a place of low self-confidence. Regardless, I attributed my emotional connection to these rides to fear, convincing others I was worried about potentially flying out of the ride or getting stuck in the middle of a giant vertical loop.

It was only when I was seventeen I finally allowed one of my best friends, Teddy, to drag me on The Incredible Hulk Coaster at Universal's Islands of Adventure. We had gone to Halloween Horror Nights the night before, which left me more terrified than I had ever been in my entire life, so I figured finally riding a rollercoaster could not be any worse. As I was buckled in, I felt calm knowing how secured I was in the ride. As I smiled at my friend, I wondered what I had been fearing all this time. But when the ride was about to start, my stomach dropped. I realized my fear was not of the safety of the ride, it was the fear of the unknown. I had no idea what the next two minutes held and I wasn't sure if I was ready to experience it. But as my friend's younger sister, who at the time was in middle school and loved rollercoasters, held my hand and told me I was going to be okay (Phoebe if you're reading this, your moral support that morning is something I still cherish to this day). I embraced my fear and shouted for the entire duration of the ride, which was possibly one of the best adrenaline rushes I have ever felt.

Now you might be wondering what the point of this story was. Well, only when I was able to actually identify my emotions and what I was feeling I was truly able to embrace my fear and make the most out of my experience riding rollercoasters. In a similar manner, it is of utmost value for patients to identify and process the myriad of emotions overwhelming them throughout the process of hospital visits, tests, and pre-operative care for them to best advocate for themselves and engage in conversation with their health professionals. While providers may be able to read your symptoms off a chart and assess the biological foundations of your condition, you know your emotional health the best and must communicate that effectively and transparently to ensure the care you receive is truly the best for you.

Emotional literacy and self-care are immensely valuable at all levels of health care, from patient, to caregiver, to health professional. Through this chapter, I will explore how to develop one's emotional intelligence and the ways in which it can benefit patients and their loved ones. Part three explores strategies to mitigate compassion fatigue and professional burnout for health care providers in further detail.

A HOSPITAL WITHOUT COMPASSION IS LIKE DISNEY WITHOUT FUN

Interestingly, the parallels between the experiences of individuals in health care settings and amusement parks is not a novel concept. In *If Disney Ran Your Hospital: 9 1/2 Things You Would Do Differently*, Fred Lee draws upon his unique professional background, having served as a vice president at two major medical centers and a cast member at Walt Disney World in Orlando. He describes the importance in both spheres of changing the mentality from solely providing a service to instead providing an emotional experience in his TEDx Talk "Patient Satisfaction or Patient Experience?" For amusement parks, this involves "meeting the emotional needs of a family to have fun together," whereas for hospitals and other health care settings, the priority is "meeting the emotional needs of a family going through fear, pain, and even tragedy together."[36] In short, "A hospital without compassion is like Disney without fun."[37]

Lee illustrates the value of prioritizing emotional connection through the example of getting your blood drawn at the hospital. He provides two very similar scenarios, but the small discrepancies serve to have the greatest impact. In the first scenario, you are met by a nice phlebotomist who comes to draw your blood. Silence ensues as you watch her tie the tourniquet on your arm, making you feel nervous and weakening your pain threshold. Even the slightest adjustment feels like your skin is being ripped off. Once she is done, you are just relieved it's all over.[38]

In the second, she comes to draw your blood but notices you are nervous. She reassures you she will do her best to be gentle. As she begins making polite conversation with you, you get distracted and before you know it, the blood draw is complete. At the end, all you can think about is you want her to be your phlebotomist the next time you need a blood draw.[39]

---

36 *TEDx Talks,* "TEDxMaastricht - Fred Lee - 'Patient Satisfaction or Patient Experience?,'" April 6, 2011, video, 17:18.
37 Ibid.
38 Ibid.
39 Ibid.

Whether we realize it or not, our emotional states play a large role throughout our interactions with our health professionals, directly impacting our levels of stress and anxiety as well as our pain thresholds, which may influence our subsequent interactions with our health professionals in the future. As we look at Lee's scenario, the patient who had "Gentle Sherry" is much more likely to provide her with a more detailed account of the nature of their pain, what has been bothering them, and their previous medical history. Those who had "Normal Sherry" and did not establish as strong of a connection may have been more reserved and/or withholding of this information, even though she realistically did not do anything objectively wrong in terms of service.

Although health professionals have a degree of accountability for fostering an atmosphere in which this level of comfort and sharing can be facilitated, we must also be realistic in recognizing not every medical professional out there will be a "Gentle Sherry." They may not take as much time to ask about your day or your personal life, but that does not necessarily take away from the level of skill and expertise they have in their field to provide you with amazing care. Rather than getting hung up on finding a doctor who initiates this degree of sharing, it is helpful to initiate such sharing as a patient. If you feel your health professional is missing information about your daily life related to your health, tell it to them, regardless of how relevant it may seem. If you feel scared, it is okay to let them know you are worried, and if you are a loved one who can sense the patient's hesitancy, advocate on their behalf. If you initiate this level of transparency, it is likely your doctor will also be more transparent and engaged in the conversation and a strong provider-patient relationship can still emerge. Remember, although doctor comes before patient in "doctor-patient relationship," both sides of the hyphen are accountable for pulling their weight to foster a strong sense of rapport and trust that will maximize the likelihood of success for whichever course of treatment you both choose.

IDENTIFYING, CONFRONTING, AND EXPRESSING DIFFICULT EMOTIONS

Numerous communication barriers have been identified that often limit patients from expressing their emotions and/or concerns to their health professionals during appointments. Patients may limit the questions they ask because they do not want to come off as unintelligent, weak, or negative. In some cases, patients are truly afraid of what the actual answer to the question will be or they feel being inquisitive will make their providers see them as a burden. While these concerns are valid, they can substantially inhibit the quality of care a patient receives, especially if these claims are based off misconceptions or misinterpretations that could have been solved through open and honest communication.

One of the most important steps in being able to enhance this quality of communication from the patient perspective is to first identify what you are feeling in the moment. It could be anger at the fact your health is potentially betraying you, sadness because you may have a tough road ahead, or perhaps even frustration because you are stuck at the doctor's office with uncertainty surrounding your future, regardless of the severity of the case. Patients and caregivers alike are often overloaded with emotions, especially anxiety, during these times, which at times has been found to potentially compromise the quality of rational decision making, judgment, and cognitive processing.[40],[41],[42] It is essential to break these emotions down and identify each individual feeling to provide health professionals with the most complete picture possible to approach treatment.

On their website, Johns Hopkins All Children's Hospital outlines some basic guidelines for dealing with difficult emotions that, frankly, are valuable for patients of all ages. The first step is identifying the emotion you are feeling, which may be accompanied by certain bodily sensations such as muscle tension or feeling your face flush. It is important, however, to look beyond just identifying the feeling to understanding why you feel this way in the first place, if you want to approach addressing it. While some of these emotions may be hard to deal with or seem insignificant, you should avoid blame and rather focus on recognizing and explaining these feelings so you can better navigate yourself toward a solution.[43]

Once you have identified and processed your emotions, you can now focus on taking action so you can both express what you feel and resolve any issues that accompany it. If you feel

---

40   Desirée Kozlowski et al., "The role of emotion in clinical decision making: an integrative literature review," *BMC Medical Education* 17, 255(2017).

41   Sarah N. Garfinkel et al., "Anger in brain and body: the neural and physiological perturbation of decision-making by emotion," *Social Cognitive and Affective Neuroscience* 11, 1(2016):150-8.

42   Petko Kusev et al., "Understanding Risky Behavior: The Influence of Cognitive, Emotional and Hormonal Factors on Decision-Making under Risk," *Frontiers in Psychology* 8, 102(2017).

43   "Dealing With Difficult Emotions," Johns Hopkins Medicine, accessed October 29, 2020.

fearful for a procedure, it may be helpful to write it down in a journal or vent about it with a loved one. At the same time, it is also helpful to mention your uncertainty to your doctor, as they can often use their expertise to provide any reassuring information specific to the procedure, medication, or treatment while also providing emotional support. Additionally, it is important to lean on those around you during these times, since social support is one of the most important factors in recovery after any kind of difficult experience, medical or nonmedical. While you may be the one with the condition, you are not going through this alone and reaching out to others for help does not make you weak: it makes you human.

In a similar manner, it is crucial caregivers and loved ones recognize that while they are valuable sources of emotional support for patients, you also are human and need to take care of yourself as well. Compassion fatigue is a serious issue, which I explore in more depth during Part three, and to help your loved ones return to their best, you need to be at your best as well. It is okay to step back at times to process what is going on, to cry, and to be fearful. In addition to providing your loved ones with an outlet for emotional expression, make sure you have one of your own to maintain your well-being during these often overwhelming processes.

While at times social pressures may push us to repress our emotions, wearing your heart on your sleeve and conveying vulnerability is one of the most admirable things you can do, not just as patients or caregivers, but as human beings. By being able to identify your emotions and feelings throughout the process, you can serve as better communicators and support systems, respectively, throughout the treatment process. In the remainder of Part two, I will go into depth on some of the more specific ways in which both patients and caregivers can embrace their curiosity and advocate for themselves in health care settings.

CHAPTER 5

GOING UNDERCOVER AS AN EXPECTING MOTHER: FROM *KARAN* TO *KAREN*

One of my favorite memories during elementary and middle school (back when homework was only a single sheet of math problems and maybe five pages of reading) was watching basketball with my parents in our living room. My mother, a passionate Miami Heat fan, would scream at the TV while my dad would laugh on the couch. While my favorite hobby was playing the newest Pokémon game on my Nintendo DS, I loved taking breaks to watch my city's home team take on the best of the best, whether from the comfort of our apartment or American Airlines Arena.

A particular game that still stands out to me was during the 2011 NBA Playoffs, when the Heat faced the Dallas Mavericks in the championship round. With the Mavericks having won three games and the Heat having won only two, the team needed to win this next game or they were out of the running for the championship. At the half, things were close as the Heat trailed behind by two points. While I don't remember a lot of the game's details other than the fact we sadly lost that night as the Mavericks were crowned champions, I do have a very distinct memory of the Miami Heat dancers, but not for the reason you might think.

While the dancers lit up the stage with an energetic and skillful performance at halftime, I was immensely struck by how their smiles and confidence never wavered. Even as our chances at victory continued to slip away from us as the Mavericks strengthened their lead, not a single dancer looked like they had lost hope in our team. Regardless of whether we won or lost a game, the Miami Heat dancers symbolized the flare and exuberance of Miami culture and the faith and love we had for our basketball team.

In many ways, the strength and positivity these dancers reflected, even at their team's hardest times, represents the role we want to serve when our loved ones are facing challenges with their health. Whether it be a family member, a close friend, or someone you just really care about, you feel that strong desire to help them fight whatever condition they face, but simultaneously recognize your overall powerlessness in terms of curing them medically. All you can do is hold their hand and plaster a smile on your face, assuring them everything will be okay, when in reality, you may have more questions than answers.

I tremendously appreciated the company of my parents and loved ones throughout my medical procedures and found their support immensely helpful in the recovery process. However, one of the moments in which I truly recognized the value of having a strong network of support throughout any medical process was during my experience as an expecting mother.

FROM *KARAN* TO *KAREN*
For those of you who flipped back to a page to reread that last sentence, let me assure you, you did not read it incorrectly. You may be wondering how a male, second-year student had any experiences related to being an expecting mother. Well, I'd love to tell you a story.

During an early meeting with my developmental editor, I talked to her about how I had reached a brick wall in my writing process. While I had some more research I wanted to do and more personal experiences I wanted to share, I was missing that spark I felt while writing some of these other stories. I needed something new: a game changer that would help me get back on track.

While we talked about potential health professionals to interview other than doctors or nurses, she suggested I talk to some doulas. Having never heard of the profession before, I was intrigued upon learning how expecting families hire these trained professionals to provide mothers with physical and emotional support, as well as information both through and beyond the process of childbirth. As DONA International (formerly Doulas of North America) beautifully summarizes their role, "Like travel guides in a foreign country, birth and postpartum doulas help support new families through the life changing experience of having a baby."[44]

---

44   DONA International, "What Is a Doula?," accessed September 07, 2020.

With the topic of childbirth in mind, I remembered how many hospitals offered classes to teach expecting parents about various aspects of pregnancy and important skills, such as Lamaze breathing and how to properly swaddle and burp your baby. Given the unsafe atmosphere of medical settings during the pandemic, I noticed many hospitals, practices, and organizations were offering these classes virtually through Zoom. As a college student who has taken classes online for the last few months, I also knew how easy it was to join a Zoom session without ever having to speak or show your face, a feature I found tremendously useful during many early morning calls.

While we originally discussed reaching out to those facilitating these classes as many instructors have previous experience as a nurse or doula, an even better idea popped into my head: what better way to learn about health education than to experience it as a student? My developmental editor laughed at my idea to pose as an expecting mother and attend these classes to investigate different health education modalities, but we decided to touch base the following week with updates.

Having been a former thespian during parts of middle and high school, I remembered the importance of "becoming" your role. I had to create a character for myself and immerse myself in it completely so I could truly understand the mindset of a patient, especially a mother now responsible for carrying another human life inside of her.

Thus, I was reborn as Karen Mirchandani. Karen is an aspiring screenwriter living with her high school sweetheart in a small loft in Tribeca. Her husband, a columnist for *The New York Times*, has been especially busy over the last few months writing articles and conducting interviews about the political aspects of the pandemic and its potential implications for the recent election. However, they have both been writing from home and are excited to welcome their first child after the next seven months. While Karen has been told her pregnancy is going well and the baby is healthy, she and her husband both have limited knowledge of the medical system, so they are currently looking for a doula to help guide them through the process.

After my backstory was complete, I signed up for multiple pregnancy related classes, ranging from more general overviews of the process of childbirth to ones specifically addressing the implications of COVID-19 on available services and changes in protocol. In these classes, I sought to analyze both the methods in which information was provided to expectant mothers and the information itself, common questions mothers had during the journey of pregnancy, and most importantly, the qualities I should be seeking in my doula.

THE VALUE OF SOCIAL SUPPORT

During her second pregnancy, Lin had never felt more alone and defeated. With one toddler already running around the house and her husband working full time at their restaurant, she did not experience much social contact with anyone. "The only interactions I had with people were with the strangers across the street fighting over parking," she said.[45]

This sense of isolation was further exacerbated when it came time for her child to be born. One Sunday night, she began

---

45   *TEDx Talks,* "What the Right Support Can Do For You: A Doula is More Than a Good Friend | Lin Liang | TEDxCUNY," May 14, 2019, video, 12:51.

experiencing contractions and spent twenty-four hours in the hospital, only to be sent home the following day because her baby was not ready for delivery. However, she returned again on Tuesday as her doctor said her baby was suddenly primed to come out. At the time, she was greeted by the hospital's doula, a sweet woman who asked how she could support Lin throughout this process. While Lin appreciated her thought, she politely declined the doula's services, thinking to herself, "I did it once. I could do it again."[46]

Unfortunately, she recognized later she really should have taken the doula's offer, as the subsequent journey leading to her child's birth was a stressful one. As she describes in her TEDx Talk "What the Right Support Can Do For You: A Doula is More Than a Good Friend," her hesitancy to unnaturally accelerate her child's birth as per her physician's recommendation was interpreted by her medical professionals as irresponsible and dangerous to the life of her unborn child. Despite her uncertainty and fear of the overwhelming situation, her doctor broke her water without her consent, which still failed to induce labor. Her doctor recommended Lin to utilize artificial chemicals to stimulate contractions, but when she and her husband asked for a minute to think about this decision, her doctor questioned her by saying, "Well, you don't want a C-section, do you?"[47]

Despite the stress and anxiety she experienced during this situation and the risk of having a preterm birth, Lin was fortunate to have given birth to a healthy baby girl. While

---

46   Ibid.

47   Ibid.

she found solace in that her daughter was born healthy and happy, she could not get over the negative aspects of the system through which women and families welcome their babies into this world, leading her to a new career path where she could become the support she lacked.

"If I told you there's a drug that can decrease the time of labor, lessen or diminish the pain of contractions, and give you a higher rate of natural delivery without complications, would you take it?"[48]

While this medication sadly does not exist, Lin happily explained while there is no drug, there are doulas who work hard to find the right resources and evidence-based information to support mothers physically and mentally throughout the often-overwhelming process of labor. By providing continuous and personalized support, doulas can even help stimulate the release of oxytocin in the mother's body, the "love hormone" which can tremendously improve the quality of labor.

Lin's story, among those of many other mothers I met throughout my various classes, made me realize the immense value of social support. When I enrolled in one specific class on giving birth during the pandemic, I expected many questions to be asked about what safety protocols would be utilized to ensure the protection of both the mother and her child. However, I was immensely surprised by the nature of some of the mothers' concerns.

---

48   Ibid.

I remember one mother frantically asking the instructor not about safety protocols, but about what clothes she should pack for her child, given no one else could bring any clothes because of restrictions on visitors. As she swiftly listed about twenty different clothing combinations (including a t-shirt and shorts, t-shirt and pants, long-sleeve and shorts, long-sleeve, shorts, and a sweatshirt, pajamas, and many more I have forgotten at this point) I couldn't help but stare incredulously at my computer screen. *How is it that this mother is so worried about clothes among the number of complications associated with pregnancy?* Luckily, no one could see my reaction given that Karen's camera and microphone were "broken," but she was happy to chime in via the Zoom chat whenever she had any questions.

Our instructor was very understanding, informing her she only needed to pack one pair of clothes the baby could leave with, given that they tremendously enjoy being swaddled in only a hospital blanket after birth. While I was initially unaffected by this interaction, it was interesting to notice the gratitude and calmness that immediately took over the expecting mother's voice. I simply realized the act of addressing one concern, while it may seem minuscule in the grand scheme of things, can make a substantial impact on an individual's mindset.

Although it is extremely important to respect the autonomy of the patient and not make their negative experience into something all about you, it is important to remember we can all play valuable roles in helping our loved ones advocate for themselves throughout their care. It could be something as simple as accompanying them to a routine checkup for moral support, holding their hand while they get an injection, or helping them research their condition and facilitate discussions of treatment options for their doctors. Regardless of the size of your contribution, they will appreciate having a solid support system to get them through whatever challenges they face.

Aside from the fascinating descriptions of the use of nitrous oxide (laughing gas) and sterile water injections in the lower back to decrease the pain of childbirth (the latter of which Karen will definitely be requesting during her birth at either Stony Brook University Hospital or Mount Sinai Hospital), I found the most valuable lesson from my birthing classes to be the importance of having someone who will accompany you every step of the way, answer all the little questions, and celebrate your accomplishments. As I asked (well, typed) my question about what qualities I should seek in my doula, the instructor summed it up in a perfect way:

"When selecting your doula, choose someone you are comfortable spending a lot of time with and spending time with naked."

As she and many of the other women reminisced about how fantastic and supportive their doulas are, I realized to be the best personal cheerleader for anyone, you have to foster an environment of love, encouragement, and most of all, acceptance. The patient cannot feel afraid to ask a question, no matter how stupid it may sound, nor should they be judged for it. While I still laugh at the regular emails I receive with Zoom invitations to join the biweekly "Circle of Mothers," I am comforted to know this community of women who are still strangers to me welcome Karen with open arms, ready to help her find the doula of her dreams.

CHAPTER 6

MEDICINE AS A TEAM SPORT PART I: FINDING FAITH IN FANTASY

––––––

"You're something of a medical mystery," my ENT told me as he observed the peculiar bump behind my left ear. I had noticed it months ago while looking in the mirror and my parents and I decided to see a specialist to hopefully identify what the strange mass was. My doctor told me he had never seen anything like it before, proceeding to call in three other specialists from the department to assist with the examination.

One would think four physicians in a room focused on your health and determining the best course of action would be comforting. For me, however, this sense of security was quickly replaced by confusion and alarm. Rather than feeling assured, I instead tried to process the medical jargon being thrown around the physicians as they speculated what the mass could be.

"Cyst, abscess, a tumor maybe?" one physician said to the others. The last possibility struck me with fear. It wouldn't be until a few months later in my ninth grade biology and biomedical science classes I would learn of the difference between a benign tumor and a malignant one. At the time, the only thing I knew was tumors are associated with cancer. I was terrified and didn't possess the knowledge to comprehend all of this information being thrown at me.

Fortunately, four MRIs and a CT scan in the following weeks determined I had an arteriovenous malformation, or AVM for short. An AVM is a tangle of blood vessels typically found in the brain, but due to its abnormal location behind my ear, it proved to have a much better prognosis. I was redirected to a craniofacial surgeon who would block the blood supply to the mass to stop it from growing and remove it. As he explained these procedures, I felt much more relaxed, as my classes had allowed me to better understand the vocabulary he was using and trust his skills and judgment.

Interestingly, my parents did not share this opinion. As I've recounted the experience with my mother, she's shared her anger and frustration about my surgeon's quick explanations without much room for questions. Not having the same passion for science and medicine as I did, she was still confused by everything we were told and had many unanswered questions. While I felt comforted by my physician's confidence and brevity, it made him appear unapproachable to my parents, leaving them with more fear than reassurance.

Although the surgery was very successful and I continue to live a happy and healthy life, I still remember the fear and uncertainty I went through while in the hospital and the confusion both myself and especially my parents felt in numerous instances. Had I not had a strong interest in health or the opportunity to take biomedical science classes early on, I probably would've remained in that same confused, insecure state I originally was in. And even with that background, there are times where I was still baffled and overwhelmed by the complex medical vocabulary and information I had to process throughout appointments and my hospitalization. Through this experience, I learned the immense value of embracing a curious approach as a patient and viewing medicine as a team sport.

USING INEXPERIENCE TO MY ADVANTAGE

A hobby I look forward to every fall is fantasy football. I was originally thrust into this world when my cousins needed an extra person for their league and asked me to join. Given my lack of knowledge and interest in football, I was initially confused by their offer, but understood very quickly after they quipped I would be an easy defeat. Intrigued by the process and determined to prove them wrong, I accepted their offer and ultimately placed second overall in the league, much to everyone's surprise. As I reflect on my sudden entrance into the realm of sports analytics, statistics, and, of course, playful trash talk, I've noticed some surprising parallels to my health-related experiences, especially as a patient.

Similar to my appointment with my ENT to diagnose my arteriovenous malformation, my introduction to fantasy football left me overwhelmed, to say the least. After agreeing to join the league, my cousins and I decided to discuss the logistics of the league.

"Should we do standard scoring or PPR?" one of my cousins asked.

"Obviously standard. Who even does PPR?" my other cousin quipped. "Ok, so it looks like our draft will be sometime in the next two weeks. We'll be doing a snake draft, of course, and no carryovers during bye weeks (these are weeks where certain teams don't play, as I would later find out after a panicked Google search). Does that sound good to everyone?"

My other cousins nodded in unison and immediately began doing practice drafts and formulating six versions of their ideal team. While I smiled and nodded as well, all I could hear were alarms signaling I was way in over my head. How was I supposed to prove myself to them when I didn't even know what PPR was? After voraciously typing the acronym into Google, I learned it meant points per reception, which prompted me to look up what exactly constituted a reception.

If you couldn't tell already, I had no idea what I was doing. During PE football, I played center because snapping the ball to the quarterback was the only thing I knew how to do. Whenever my dad would tell me to watch the Super Bowl, I would sneak into my bedroom to play the latest Pokémon game on my Nintendo DS, claiming I had homework but he should call me whenever the commercials started. Although I was a water polo athlete and enthralled by the camaraderie, aggression, and excitement in the world of sports, football was never appealing to me.

Here I was, in a room filled with experts in a field completely unfamiliar to me and who spoke a completely different language but expected me to make crucial decisions about my team, without taking the time to explain any of the rules or terminology. Does this sound like a story you've heard before? The feelings of anxiety, confusion, and uncertainty I felt in those moments of the draft directly paralleled those I felt during my doctor's appointment years prior. Of course, hearing my cousins laugh about PPR brought about much less stress than my doctors casually suggesting I may have a tumor, but I still felt helpless and uncertain about my future. Overwhelmed by all of the information presented to me, I found it easier to smile and nod, rather than take the initiative to fully understand what was going on around me so I could make informed decisions in the best interests of my team.

This tendency to be passive in the face of adversity is something many patients may experience. When faced with the intricate lexicon of the medical field coupled with the storm of emotions going through your mind as your doctor describes your diagnosis and treatment options, it is natural to feel confused and overwhelmed. Information, especially about your health and well-being, takes time to be processed and fully understood. The naturally complex nature of medical terminology makes this even more difficult, even for those trained in these fields.

However, if I learned anything from the world of fantasy football and from my experiences as a patient, it is that curiosity, (while difficult to express at times) and a willingness to accept the unknown are essential to navigating such novel situations. While I learned a lot about fantasy football independently, I also learned very quickly approaching the league like a researcher would not help me become a competitive player. While I was trying to build football literacy through research, my cousins had built it through experience, something that had proved to be much more valuable. For them, this was a way of life: a language they had developed fluency in through constant practice and passion.

During my first league, I was able to skate by with a few early wins using the videos I watched and looking at the predicted statistics. But eventually, my beginner's luck faded and I entered a terrible losing streak that exposed my fundamental lack of experience and understanding. My cousins tried to engage me in trades, in reality, could have benefitted the both of us. But my confusion and suspicion prevented me from capitalizing on such opportunities, resulting in their teams becoming stronger and mine failing to catch up.

I soon realized I needed a game plan of my own if I wanted to prove myself as a worthy competitor: I was not some joke that had just joined to meet the requirement of participants. It was at that point I took a step back and analyzed the situation. To my cousins, my weakness was I did not understand football: I never really watched the games, could not comprehend much of the terminology, and frankly, lacked the same passion and general interest they had. I was not perceived to be a threat.

However, this experience perpetuated a lesson I carry throughout my life, especially as a water polo player:

"Every weakness contains within itself a strength."

— SHŪSAKU ENDŌ

My inexperience in the realm of fantasy football suddenly became my competitive edge. Because my cousins never saw me as a threat, they were very willing to give me advice on how to best set up my team to perform well each week. They assumed that regardless of how much help I received, I would still never be able to outsmart them. That was where they were wrong.

Rather than pitting my football knowledge against my adversaries, I would use my inexperience as a facade while the experience of those helping me strengthened my team's performance. My game plan involved collecting important information about how to win while simultaneously pitting my opponents against each other, essentially doing most of the work for me. Instead of allowing my lack of knowledge to remain a weakness, I turned it into my greatest strength by using it to collect important knowledge from my peers and turning it against them, allowing me to improve my rank, and ultimately, place in the top three of all the leagues I have competed in.

FROM THE STADIUM TO THE SCANNER
My willingness to acknowledge my shortcomings and ask for help simultaneously served as a valuable asset throughout my experience as a patient. I remember when I saw my first physician about the strange bump behind my ear in India

the summer after I finished eighth grade. My mother and I went to a small office to meet with an otolaryngologist (ear, nose, and throat doctor) a family friend recommended to us. Many thoughts raced through my head as the doctor's cold fingers poked the mass. Is it cancer? Maybe it's nothing. Why isn't he saying anything?

After further examination, he told my mother and I the mass was probably a cyst, which was nothing to be worried about. However, he thought it would be best for me to get an MRI and an echocardiogram at the local hospital to assess the mass and ensure my heart was healthy. These were to be two short routine procedures. My mother and I thanked him and left, preparing to get my scans done the next day at the nearest hospital.

***

My mother and I entered the hospital the next day calmly, reassured by the doctor's encouraging words. *We'll be out of here in no time*, I thought. We decided to do the echocardiogram first. The monographer was very thorough and explained everything to me as she completed the scan. I remember the feeling of the warm jelly she squeezed out of the bottle that allowed the transducer to effectively send sound waves that would bounce off my heart and produce its image. She pointed out the four chambers, snapped some pictures, and told me everything looked great. I was immensely relieved and almost excited for my MRI, expecting a similar, positive experience. Little did I know what would follow would be the first of a series of uncomfortable and tedious experiences.

As I approached the large, looming machine in the radiology wing, I was immediately intrigued, but also somewhat scared. There was not much space for movement, but I figured it would not be much of a problem considering the technicians and my physician mentioned I would not be in there for long. I went to lie down and they placed a coil over my head, informing me it would take pictures of the mass. Calmly, I told them I was ready and they started the scan.

"Remember, you must stay as still as possible. Any small movement can blur the scan and we will have to start over," the radiologist reminded me.

The MRI machine suddenly made many whirring noises, indicating the scanning process had begun. At first I sat there intrigued, but quickly became annoyed by the sounds and my immobility. The whole experience was extremely uncomfortable and I eventually began feeling claustrophobic and alarmed, telling the radiologist I needed a break to move and readjust. They stopped the scan and let me stretch for a second, but proceeded to tell me sternly they needed me to stay still.

Rather than feeling comforted and supported, I instead felt annoyed. The otolaryngologist had told me the procedure would be short. But what I had forgotten was time is relative: for a physician who conducts surgeries that usually run for hours, a fifteen-to-forty-five-minute scan sounds like a walk in the park. But for a nervous, fidgety teenager, an immobilizing scan with only whirring sounds for entertainment felt like a year. Rather than staying still and finishing the MRI quicker, I almost wanted to move my body in defiance to what felt like a complete betrayal to my fourteen-year-old brain.

Eventually, the radiologists were able to render a good enough image and we were finally able to leave the office. While the tedious process frustrated me, I was also relieved I would probably never have to get another MRI again and hopeful these scans would be sufficient for the specialist we would eventually consult in Miami.

***

When we first met with the craniofacial surgeon who would ultimately operate on me, he informed us the MRI scans we got from India were not detailed enough for him to decide what the next best step would be. From the MRI, he deducted an alternate diagnosis; he believed the mass behind my ear was an arteriovenous malformation, a tangle of blood vessels usually found in the brain. He wanted to confirm this theory with four MRI scans, which would examine the mass from two separate angles. Two of the scans would use contrast, a dye that would better elucidate my blood vessels and brain, allowing for a clearer image.

"The scans should take about three and a half hours," he said calmly.

I let the sentence run in my head one more time. *Three and a half hours.* While I appreciated how thorough my surgeon's action plan was, I abhorred the idea of having to lie in the MRI machine again, for one, let alone four scans. I barely even lasted during the forty-five minutes of agony the last time. However, I knew it was in my best interest and was determined to go through with the scans with minimal disruption. I didn't want to let my discomfort be an inconvenience to him, my mother, or any of the other medical professionals involved.

Given the exhausting duration of these scans, my surgeon, mother, and I decided it would be in my best interest to schedule the scans that weekend at six in the morning so I could sleep through them. In retrospect, I should have known this was not going to work. As a side sleeper, lying on my back felt really uncomfortable, which, coupled with the charmingly awful whirring of the machine, did not make falling asleep any easier. However, the immense fatigue from waking up at five in the morning eventually did its job.

About two hours into the examination, I woke up, dazed and uncertain of where I was. I had completely forgotten I was having an MRI scan. Scared out of my mind, I squeezed the panic button ten times, causing the technicians to immediately roll me out of the machine and stop the second scan midway, meaning we had to start the second scan all over again before they could even inject me with the contrast for the third and fourth.

At that point, I was done trying to be the perfect patient. It was clear my efforts to be stoic were only making the whole process difficult for all parties involved, especially myself. I informed the radiologist I was extremely uncomfortable in the machine and without any entertainment, I would not be able to stay still for three and a half hours. After some deliberation, my radiologist offered my mother and I the option of sedating me with anesthesia so I would be unconscious throughout the entire process. While anesthetizing me was not ideal, I burst with joy at the idea and immediately agreed. A week later, I remember counting down from ten. The next time I suddenly woke up, I was greeted with the smiling face of my mother telling me all four scans were completed and were the clearest images yet.

PRACTICING WHAT I PREACH

It was through this experience I realized it was not my job as a patient to please my medical professionals or even my mother. Because I tried to be this perfect and compliant patient and resisted my discomfort, I ended up making the experience frustrating for everyone involved, even though we were all on the same team. While I hated the idea of being selfish, it was only when I put my needs first and asked my doctors for other options we were able to find what was in my best interest and allowed for my successful surgery. Asking questions and expressing discomfort were not signs of weakness. Rather, they were assets that strengthened our action plan and facilitated my successful prognosis.

When it comes to your health care and your medical decisions, you have to remember YOU are the patient. While it is natural to want to please authority figures and avoid being a burden, it is YOUR health on the line. As patients, we have to be comfortable with being selfish and communicating how we feel. If there is something you are not comfortable with, don't be afraid to ask for other options. Had I not asked if there were alternate means to get the scan, I never would have been offered the sedation that allowed the radiologist to develop the clear MRI, which confirmed my surgeon's diagnosis and provided him with the proper visualization for the successful removal of my AVM.

When approaching conversations with your health professionals, it is important to remember you're both on the same team and share a common goal. By approaching situations with curiosity and respect and voicing your concerns, you and your providers can work together to create the best game plan for your care. Instead of trying to be a perfect patient, focus on being a curious patient and a strong self-advocate, the qualities of a true MVP.

PART III

USING CURIOSITY
TO CURE THE CAT

CHAPTER 7

MEDICINE AS A TEAM SPORT PART II: TURNING FANTASY INTO REALITY

———

In Chapter six, I discussed the surprising parallels between my experiences as a patient and as a fantasy football player, highlighting the merits of viewing medicine as a team sport. To provide some more actionable advice for patients to advocate for themselves, I will continue to explore this metaphor while simultaneously providing the narratives of other patients who have used facets of this mindset to enhance their care.

RECRUITING YOUR TEAM

When assembling your team for fantasy sports or even as a coach of a real team, many factors go into selecting the best athletes, including performance statistics, work ethic, and general attitude, all of which are extremely important in curating a strong, cohesive unit. While some football players may have amazing track records, they automatically become questionable picks during a fantasy draft if they are injury prone or lack compatibility with their teammates. Although this selection process is fundamentally different from picking a health professional responsible for making important judgment calls that could impact whether you live or die, a lot can be learned from its holistic and multifaceted nature.

While talking to many friends and family members regarding how they picked their medical professionals, many different factors were mentioned that shaped the decision-making process. Some valued bedside manner the most, seeking a provider who was kind, patient, and willing to slowly walk them through every step of the process. On the other hand, others preferred a confident and concise provider they could trust and have minimal interaction with unless absolutely necessary. In addition to these two approaches, some individuals only cared about whether they would be completely covered by insurance or if any trusted friends or family members already had positive experiences with them.

These conversations were eye-opening for me, allowing me to recognize the many different and valuable factors that go into selecting a provider. Throughout my own experiences as a patient, my parents were the ones who made most of the decisions regarding my physicians, valuing both bedside manner and recommendations from family friends and my long-term physicians. However, as a college student in Nashville who now has to find a new primary care physician, I realized there were even more factors I should consider when making a decision.

In a video produced by John and Hank Green for their You-Tube channel "How to Adult," Hank provides a similar breakdown of considerations for selecting a primary care physician. For example, it is important to consider your pre-existing conditions or chronic illnesses that may require special attention during annual checkups. In certain cases, specialists you may already be visiting regularly can simultaneously serve as your primary care physician, such as one's gynecologist. Another factor to consider is the space in which the provider practices. Some patients may prefer to visit doctors at smaller private offices, where they may receive more personalized care. However, others may opt to select a physician practicing directly in a hospital, where they have convenient access to certain facilities if emergencies arise and may have more flexible hours.[49]

Lastly, always make sure to do as much research as you can on prospective providers, including criteria such as how often they renew their certification, how much experience they've had, and whether they receive any funding from pharmaceutical companies to endorse certain products, and don't be afraid to have more than one backup.[50] While someone may seem to be an amazing fit on paper, it is important you go to your first appointment and evaluate the quality of their service. Saying no and seeking second opinions doesn't make you an annoying, disrespectful, or bad patient; it shows you care about your health and are focused on finding the best fit for your team as you approach the challenges ahead.

---

49   *How to Adult,* "How to Choose a Doctor (in the U.S.)," September 13, 2017, video, 4:27.
50   Ibid.

BEING CREATIVE WITH YOUR PLAYBOOK

In every team sport, it is likely your coach has a playbook detailing some of the best strategies they have discovered to emerge victorious against even the worthiest adversaries. Whether it be establishing an impenetrable defense or preparing a vigilant, creative offense that is ready for a counterattack, many teams employ a variety of plays and approaches to outsmart their opponents. However, much like any strong rival team, illnesses are vigilant and adaptive. While some strategies are extremely effective against certain teams, other opponents may adapt faster and are much more difficult to combat. In the same regard, treatment regiments against certain bacterial and viral infections, cancers, and other conditions require the same level of vigilance and creativity. Although medical professionals usually determine such approaches, patients can simultaneously participate in this process to curate the best approach for success.

I learned the power of such creativity and resilience when hearing the story of Peggy, a stage IV cancer survivor. As a woman who was never keen on drugs or alcohol and primarily ate home-cooked meals, Peggy was shocked upon receiving her diagnosis in her thirties. When I asked about her experiences through treatment, she told me she was very fortunate to have an oncologist who was honest with her. He told her while he would do everything he could on his end, the other 50 percent was up to her to find ways to embrace self-healing within her own lifestyle. Granted this new autonomy in her care coupled with her chemotherapy treatments, Peggy told me she embraced numerous unique approaches, including embedding meditation and yoga into her daily lifestyle and immersing herself in the world of nature. She told me other than her health professionals in the hospital, she found "mentors" in the trees, birds, and park benches around her, allowing her to come to terms with her diagnosis and feel an incredible sense of wellness that continues to guide her life today, especially in her role as a life coach.

While Peggy still met with her health professionals for essential treatment to combat her cancer, the autonomy and creativity she used within her own lifestyle was a crucial part in her recovery and well-being, something that should be exercised by all patients. After six months of her treatment, she has been able to rely solely on her new lifestyle to continue cultivating her wellness, embodying the power of believing in and trusting oneself. Although traditional approaches may work, it is important to approach treatment with an open mind and to seek out the treatment protocols that will be best for you. Posing such questions and bringing in research about unique approaches is not the sign of a disrespectful patient. Being proactive about your care and what is best for you is a key facet of patient self-advocacy we can all learn from, and it is important to find medical professionals who will support you through that process.

MAKING THE MOST OF EACH TEAM MEMBER'S TALENTS
As we reach early adolescence, our bodies begin to change in many mysterious ways.

While some of you readers may roll your eyes at this clichéd statement we are all told once we reach this age (trust me, I rolled my eyes while writing it), it is one of the most perfect ways to introduce teenagers to the myriad of differences they will begin to experience during this key developmental transition. As dramatic shifts in hormone levels alter our body chemistry, we begin to see ourselves getting taller, having different voices, and, perhaps my least favorite, developing acne.

At the same time, these new characteristics may also lead to the development of new sources of insecurity and anxiety, as many begin to focus more on their appearance and social circles. While students may use extracurricular involvements, socioeconomic status, or intelligence to shape their friend group, our biology suddenly becomes a new factor in the picture that influences the social food chain. As a result, it may become difficult for us to differentiate between natural, developmental changes and unnatural changes that may actually harm us.

Emily Ross was a normal teenager studying in Michigan when she noticed herself undergoing some strange physical symptoms. She began overheating very easily, had trouble sleeping and eating regularly, and began feeling anxious, jittery, and depressed.[51]

"When my parents relayed these symptoms to my doctor, they were quickly reassured that these developmental periods were naturally erratic and that my body would stabilize itself eventually."[52] As a result, she dismissed these symptoms and began internalizing them as personality traits, rather than indications of a greater problem.

"So I began to accept these symptoms as quirks. When I stopped wearing a winter jacket, I explained that I overheat easily.

---

51   *TEDx Talks,* "Emily Ross: Life or Death: The Power of Health Advocacy," June 3, 2016, video, 16:29.
52   Ibid.

When all of my friends were growing and I stayed the same height and weight throughout my teen years, I cited genetics as the culprit. When I missed weeks of school from being sick, I said that my immune system happens to be weaker than most. And when my depression began to affect my aspirations, I claimed that I was simply a pessimist."[53]

Since these symptoms gradually intensified as she developed, her body was able to adapt to them and she believed her experiences of feeling bad all the time were normal. However, they especially peaked during her sophomore year, which made it difficult for her to deal with stress and led to suicidal ideation. As a result, her parents took her to a psychiatrist, who prescribed an antidepressant and diagnosed her with multiple disorders. But to Emily, something still didn't quite add up considering how rapidly she began to spiral.[54]

Ultimately, she was saved by a routine blood test ordered by an endocrinologist, who diagnosed her with a near-fatal case of Graves' disease. Graves' disease is an auto-immune disorder that attacks the thyroid, a butterfly-shaped gland in the middle of the neck that produces hormones influencing metabolism, growth, body temperature, and many other factors. As a result of her condition, Emily's own immune system was attacking her thyroid, causing it to overproduce these hormones and resulting in her abnormal physical and psychological symptoms.[55]

---

53   Ibid.
54   Ibid.
55   Ibid.

Thanks to this diagnosis, Emily's doctors were able to prescribe her medications that would regulate her hormone levels before her condition worsened. After about a year of regular treatment, her hormone levels normalized. This, coupled with initiative she took at home and over the summer, allowed her to return to school with the rest of her class as a junior and graduate on schedule.[56]

While this experience was very difficult for Emily, she used it as a means to educate others and empower them to advocate for their health. In her TEDx Talk "Life or Death: The Power of Health Advocacy," Emily shares her story and provides many valuable suggestions for people to better advocate for themselves during medical appointments, such as taking notes during the appointment.[57]

"You know you're in there and you feel like you understand what they're saying…you're following. But as soon as you walk out, you find that you've lost most of the details."[58]

Given the average appointment lasts only fifteen minutes, it is difficult for patients to completely retain all of the complex information they are told during such a short time period, especially since they are generally not feeling well and may also feel stressed or anxious. By recording questions in advance or writing down what your medical professional says in real time, you have the opportunity to process the information later and look back at it for reference if there is any more confusion.

---

56   Ibid.
57   Ibid.
58   Ibid.

However, perhaps the most important advice she gives for health advocacy is the importance of doing due diligence on your own health prior to meeting with your doctor. This includes having a comprehensive understanding of one's family history and effectively communicating one's symptoms. While not all medical conditions are genetic, family histories can help identify trends and correlations that may lead to a proper diagnosis. Although nothing in my family medical history suggests any predisposition or trends of developing arteriovenous malformations, it appears this information may have helped Emily's doctors recognize her illness much quicker.

"I wish I had taken my family's health history more seriously. Most of the females in my family were hypothyroid while I was hyperthyroid, so while their thyroids underproduced hormone, mine overproduced, which means that we experienced opposite symptoms. I was unable to recognize this link, but my doctor was able to."[59]

As she beautifully points out, while patients may not be able to identify specific trends in their family histories on their own, doctors are trained to connect the dots and identify the patient's condition. For this reason, it is also extremely important to be as clear and specific as possible when communicating your symptoms, as this allows your medical professional to more efficiently determine the underlying problem and the best course of action.

"During your appointment when your doctor asks you how you're feeling, discuss possible health concerns as thoroughly

---

59   Ibid.

as you can...If you simply say that you had a cough, that could indicate a variety of problems. However, if you say that you've had a cough for over a month, that already directs the doctor's attention to more specific possible causes. The broad symptoms I experienced with Graves' disease did not worry many of the doctors I saw. For example, when they checked my blood pressure and noticed that my heart rate was abnormally fast, they asked me if I was nervous. Had I been more aware of my health, I could've told them that my heart was always racing, even when I was about to fall asleep. I also could've mentioned my family's health history, even if I didn't know the exact symptoms and even if those symptoms didn't sound familiar to those doctors, they still would have likely ordered me a blood test just to make sure...This might have led to an earlier diagnosis which might have led to an earlier intervention."[60]

Emily's story reminds us while health professionals have the incredible skill of diagnosing and curing individuals of their illnesses, patients also bring in crucial information and context that can accelerate and enhance the treatment process. It is important patients do their due diligence by becoming informed of their family's medical history and communicating their own symptoms as thoroughly and effectively as possible to their health professionals. Rather than letting yourself sit on the sidelines, jump off the bench and become a part of the conversation so you and your health care provider can best maximize your chances of victory against whatever "adversary" you may face.

---

60   Ibid.

HAVING FAITH IN YOUR TEAM

Throughout this chapter, I have included various techniques to increase one's autonomy and involvement within their own care, whether within the process of selecting a professional or the process of selecting a treatment method. However, it is also important to remember the importance of trusting your team at the end of the day. Lean on your loved ones and your health professionals to support you throughout this process because you are not alone. After you curate the right team of individuals who respect your perspectives and act in your best interests, it is important you believe in their experience, skills, and love because at the end of the day, none of them will want to see you in pain. At times, it is important to let yourself step back and let your team play the game: after all, they're your top picks and will do whatever they can to support you.

GOOD QUESTIONS TO ASK YOUR HEALTH PROFESSIONAL DURING AN APPOINTMENT

- **What are my options?**
- **What are the short-term and long-term outcomes of this procedure/treatment/approach?**
- **What impacts will this course of action have on my career and lifestyle?** It is important to be as specific as possible about your individual situation, as this could impact which course of action you ultimately pursue.
- **What will happen if I decide to do nothing at all?** This may seem like an unintelligent question but it can actually provide valuable insight regarding the urgency of your situation and if taking more time to explore other options is viable.
- **Will this service be covered by my insurance?**

- **What are possible scenarios and timelines that may result from this approach?**
- **How does my family history influence my risk for certain conditions?** If possible, it would be beneficial to get a copy of your family history and/or records so you are always prepared to present future health professionals with this important information.
- **Honestly Doc, I'm really scared about ____. Can we talk about this a little more in depth?** If something is really troubling you, no matter how minuscule, you most definitely should articulate this fear so your health professional can help talk you through it.
- **What are the best resources for me to do my own research and learn more about my diagnosis?**

Lastly, and perhaps the most important question you can ask:

- **Any other question you have!** When it comes to your health and your life, there is no such thing as a stupid question. It is important you articulate any and all concerns you have so you can approach the road ahead with confidence and develop a strong sense of trust in the treatment plan you and your health care provider decide is best.

CHAPTER 8

PAGING DR. GOOGLE

It was a bright, sunny day in Miami, as most days are throughout the year when the rain isn't violently pouring. I remember sitting at our kitchen island, doing my calculus homework while munching on some Oreo Thins (the new "healthy snack" I decided to add to my diet), when my brother Kabir walked in with a look of concern and shock.

"Guys, my pee is brown!"

My mother and I glanced at each other in confusion, certain he was either pulling a prank on us or just overexaggerating. He proceeded to explain how he had googled "brown pee" and came across a diagnosis of rhabdomyolysis, a rare exercise complication that occurs when muscle cells burst and leak their contents into the bloodstream, leaving one at high risk for severe kidney damage. Some of the symptoms included muscle weakness and dehydration, which he had definitely been experiencing, but nothing like he had previous felt even after some of his most strenuous workouts. I had generally been apprehensive about self-diagnosis using the Internet, especially because the last time I had googled the reasons for a stomachache, the options ranged from a stomach virus to a tumor. But for some weird reason, I had a feeling Kabir wasn't joking this time.

My mom, on the other hand, was not convinced and handed him a cup to pee in so she could see for herself. After a quick bottle of water, Kabir returned back with a cup of liquid that looked like it came straight out of a fountain drink machine and was left to sit for an hour after the ice melted. Now believing something didn't seem right, my mom and dad drove Kabir to the emergency room, sure it was harmless and his soreness was just from trying to flex a little too hard at the gym.

Later, we'd find out Kabir was, in fact, correct. The emergency physician who had examined him told my parents he'd caught it just in time. If he'd came in even a couple hours later, he could've risked severe internal damage that could have created the need to remove one of his kidneys. The medical professionals quickly hooked him up to an IV he would need for two weeks to flush out his bloodstream and reported he could not exercise for the next two months to avoid further damage, much to his dismay. Luckily, however, he recovered quickly and is in astounding health as we speak.

While my family and friends still joke about the story of Kabir's brown pee and the two-pound pink dumbbells he was forced to use as he eased his way back into the world of exercise, this experience reminded me of the value the Internet can have in medical treatment. As I briefly explored in Part one, recent technological innovations coupled with the current global climate have made the Internet omnipresent in the health sphere, constantly changing the way we approach medical care from all roles and providing immediate educational resources at our fingertips. However, despite such benefits, the Internet is simultaneously capable of spreading misinformation and creating paranoia if used irresponsibly, making it a double-edged sword that must be wielded carefully. Given its increased role in our daily lives and health care as a whole, especially in the context of the pandemic, I will use this chapter to explore how this double-edged sword can become the most powerful weapon in your arsenal if used responsibly and effectively.

WHO IS "DR. GOOGLE?"
In many ways, the Internet serves as a very convenient resource for people seeking health-related information. It provides quick, easy results with just the click of a button while also creating a sense of anonymity that allows individuals to pose questions they might feel uncomfortable asking a health professional directly. By having easy access to this information, patients can feel empowered to advocate for themselves and create opportunities for active involvement in discourse surrounding their diagnoses and treatment plans.

However, while this almost unlimited access to resources is immensely beneficial, it can also be extremely overwhelming, especially for those with limited health literacy or knowledge of medical terminology. As a result, certain individuals may find themselves very preoccupied with constantly monitoring their health through such resources, conducting searches on every symptom they experience. This, in turn, may lead to a general sense of fear and paranoia surrounding one's health as well as distrust of the health care industry at large, especially if their findings and ultimate diagnosis do not corroborate.

In fact, such negative consequences attributed to the increased fixation on Internet resources for purposes of self-diagnosis has led to the development of a concept known as *cyberchondria*. While the term's origins do not appear grounded in the field of mental health, but rather in sensationalist journalism, it has become increasingly referred to as an actual disorder.[61]

As defined by certified cognitive behavioral therapy practitioner Coach Simona in her podcast *Simplify Your Life*, cyberchondria is "the unfounded escalation of concerns about common symptomology based on the review of search results in literature online."[62] During her podcast episode, she discusses her own tribulations with cyberchondria and advice she applies to her daily life to help those who are facing similar challenges, such as reframing your negative thought patterns through cognitive behavioral therapy strategies, taking time for introspection to truly understand your body, and, if your symptoms continue to escalate, seeing a medical professional.

"Ever since I was a little kid…I was always on the lookout for something that was wrong with my health. And I always fixated on the thought that I was sick. Then, came the Internet and took it to the next level. Now, I had a partner in crime and that partner in crime was called Google."[63]

---

61 Vladan Starcevic, David Berle, and Sandra Arnáez, "Recent Insights Into Cyberchondria," *Current Psychiatry Reports* 22, 11(2020):56.

62 Coach Simona, "Episode 41: Obsessed with Googling Symptoms? Meet Cyberchondria," March 19, 2019, in *Simplify Your Life*, podcast, MP3 audio, 06:42.

63 Ibid.

HOW TO BEST CONSULT "DR. GOOGLE" FOR YOUR HEALTH NEEDS

While cyberchondria may prove to be a serious public health issue, I am by no means trying to suggest casually using the Internet to monitor one's health equates to having a condition; rather, I wanted to elucidate some of the potential harms that arise from being overwhelmed by the plethora of medical information available from the Internet.

It has become increasingly common to consult "Dr. Google" for information regarding one's health. According to statistics related to customer trends in health care released by Doctor. com in 2018, "Approximately 80% of survey respondents have used the internet to make a health care-related search in the past year," whether it be related to symptoms they are experiencing or in the pursuit of finding a healthcare provider.[64] While the use of online health resources is not necessarily an issue, it is important to ensure individuals are conducting this practice responsibly and in their best interests.

I myself will openly admit to irresponsibly using search engines at times to avoid walking to the student health center. During the fall semester of my freshman year, there were definitely weeks where I felt under the weather but refused to make the trip to see a health care provider because I was "too busy" studying for my midterm exams and writing papers. Instead, I consulted "Dr. Google" and found myself popping cough drops like candy, rubbing copious amounts of Vicks VapoRub on my neck to "cure" my sore throat, and preparing

---

64   "2018 Customer experience trends in healthcare," Doctor.com, accessed on February 05, 2021.

every home remedy possible to alleviate my symptoms, proud of myself for handling my health concerns.

Feeling a sense of triumph, I called my parents with excitement to tell them of my recent successes. Instead, they berated me for prioritizing my academic endeavors over my physical and emotional well-being, reminding me while they wanted me to do well in my classes, no grade was worth compromising my health. While I still admit to falling into this trap occasionally during particularly difficult weeks where I also happen to feel slightly sick, I have begun to prioritize my health, starting with seeking advice from websites more reputable than the *wikiHow* article "How to Treat and Prevent a Common Cold" and visiting a health professional if my symptoms continue to progress.

To present you with the best advice for using online resources to navigate and advocate for your health, here are some of the best tips I gathered through research and a wonderful conversation with Dr. John Bradford Hill, a hand and upper extremity surgeon and assistant professor of plastic surgery at the Vanderbilt University Medical Center.

AVOID USING THE INTERNET AS A TOOL FOR SELF-DIAGNOSIS.
While tempting to jump to conclusions based on the immense amount of information available, which can sometimes lead to important discoveries (look at Kabir's story!), the Internet should not be a substitute for visiting a health care provider, whether it be your primary care physician, nurse practitioner, or a physician assistant. In an Australian study evaluating the quality of various free online symptom checking tools, the researchers explain while these sources

are useful, "Diagnosis is not a single assessment, but rather a process requiring knowledge, research, clinical examination and testing, and the passage of time, impossible to replicate in a single online interaction."[65]

That being said, there is no harm in doing some preliminary research regarding your symptoms so the knowledge gap is less of a factor when you finally have a conversation with your health professional. Just don't commit yourself to one condition or one course of action until you know for sure your diagnosis is, in fact, your diagnosis.

CONSULT ONLINE RESOURCES *AFTER* YOU RECEIVE A DIAGNOSIS FROM A HEALTH PROFESSIONAL.

According to Dr. Hill, one of the most effective ways to use the Internet as a tool to enhance your health is approaching online sources following your diagnosis. Prior to a consultation, there is much more uncertainty surrounding your unique situation, giving your mind the freedom to explore the worst possibilities and making you more prone to panicking about what could be a very manageable condition. Rather, it is more useful to return to a search engine after a conversation with a health professional and a diagnosis in mind, which will narrow your search to targeted resources specific to your situation. For example, if a patient who initially presents with a headache is diagnosed with having a migraine with aura, they can seek out specific resources regarding medications, treatments, and lifestyle changes to mitigate their symptoms, rather than having to look through every

---

65   Michella G. Hill, Moira Sim, and Brennen Mills, "The quality of diagnosis and triage advice provided by free online symptom checkers and apps in Australia," *The Medical Journal of Australia* 212, 11(2020):514-519.

single resource dealing with all headaches. Be as specific as possible when conducting these searches to save yourself time and find the best information available for you.

SEEK OUT REPUTABLE ONLINE RESOURCES.
While the specificity of your search criteria is important, you should always be mindful of where you get your information from. For example, the source of a website's funding is directly apparent in their URL. Websites ending in ".gov" are funded by the government, others ending in ".edu" are maintained by educational institutions, and noncommercial organizations typically end in ".com" and ".org." In terms of seeking the most reputable sources, websites with governmental and educational funding sources tend to be the best, although there are definitely great ones ending in ".com" and ".org." It's equally as important to be mindful of the source credentials. Additionally, numerous foundations associated with specific conditions can provide valuable support and guidance for future steps.

CREATE AND MAINTAIN A "HEALTHCARE RESUME."
With the increased prevalence of electronic medical records (EMRs), medical information has become more consolidated and accessible to consumers. For this reason, Dr. Hill recommends patients strive to maintain a "healthcare resume," consisting of a patient's health care providers, medical history, and current medications, rather than just bringing in some bottles of medications they are taking. By doing so, any new physicians who hop onto your case will be well versed in your specific situation and know who to consult to optimize your medical care. If you do not have immediate access to such information, I strongly recommend you reach out to

your primary care provider and request your medical history to better educate yourself and create opportunities to find the appropriate resources online.

PURSUE CHANNELS THAT OFFER SOCIAL SUPPORT.
Given the emotionally overwhelming toll of being a patient, even individuals with the most physicians and specialists on their cases often feel alienated due to their conditions, especially for chronic ones. For this reason, it is valuable to use the Internet to seek out support groups (Facebook ones are pretty common) consisting of other individuals and their loved ones who have a similar condition. Not only can these groups provide opportunities to make new friends, but they can also help you learn and connect with others by listening to their individual stories rife with both success and turbulence. And if you ever feel ready, the platforms such groups offer would be incredible to share your own life experiences, which may help another person in a similar situation find their way through it.

TAKE EVERYTHING YOU READ ON THE INTERNET WITH A GRAIN OF SALT.
Remember your body is unlike any other in existence. Each person's biology is influenced by genetic and environmental factors, meaning conditions and illnesses can manifest themselves in different ways for each individual. For this reason, it is important to be mindful much of the health information on the Internet is reflective of the experiences of the majority of individuals with certain conditions. This is why it is especially important to be in contact with a health care provider if you feel something is wrong as they are better equipped than any search engine to determine your diagnosis and the best course of action for you.

Additionally, be mindful many online sources provide an entire spectrum of potential conditions that may match your symptoms, from minor infections to life-threatening diseases, which is why many see it as a double-edged sword. However, if you know what to expect and go in prepared to responsibly use these resources, you can turn "Dr. Google" into one of the most powerful weapons in your arsenal.

CHAPTER 9

KAREN REVISITED: THE CHEERLEADING DAYS

——

To provide some more actionable advice for individuals seeking to support their loved ones through health challenges, I would like to return to my alias Karen's experiences I detailed in Chapter six. As I sat through these classes while drinking some iced coffee and taking notes on the complicated yet beautiful journey of having a child, many thoughts raced through my head:

- *Karen is a strong, independent woman and the skills and information she has learned from these classes will be valuable assets in allowing her to feel empowered to speak up throughout her medical care.*
- *While the idea of an undisturbed birth is immensely appealing, the unsolicited demonstration of a woman giving birth to her child in a kiddie pool in the middle of her living room was not persuasive enough for Karen to consider that as a birthing option. However, we both definitely respect the*

woman in the video for advocating for the birthing modality that fits her needs the best.

- *If doulas are so amazing for pregnant women, why aren't there more roles like this in other specialties?*

The last one is definitely a thought that has stuck with me for a while (other than the occasional flashback to the live water birth). The idea of implementing additional social support in the form of a social worker or health advocate is not one that is, by any means, novel. Many patients have found value in simply having someone who is available to help them understand the complex lexicon and physiological mechanisms that surround their diagnoses and empower them to facilitate meaningful conversations with their health professionals. However, the idea of having a social worker accompany a patient for a major operation or important checkup does not seem as commonplace as having a doula accompany a pregnant woman to an appointment with her OB/GYN, despite their similar value in other specialties.

THE UNIVERSAL DOULA APPROACH

To illustrate the value of advocates, I'd like to share the story of Brad Lewis, a fifty-seven-year-old Caucasian psychiatric and medical humanities professor at New York University. I came across this story when reading a paper he wrote along with Annie Robinson and Danielle Spencer titled "Illness Doula: Adding a New Role to Healthcare Practice." Brad's journey through the health care system began at the optometrist's office when he went to get a new prescription for his glasses. The optometrist, unable to correct his vision with glasses, suggested he see an ophthalmologist to check for cataracts and gave him the name of a physician who she had not met, but was "sure he was nice."[66]

Unsatisfied, he did some research "looking for an ophthalmologist who seemed like he or she might have a decent bedside manner—most of what I had to go on were those questionable internet rating sites and the few physicians who had pictures."[67] Upon finding one, he was diagnosed with cataracts but was disappointed by the physician's disinterest in discussing future steps; he was only provided with a home test that involved him consistently looking at a fixed point because if he ultimately could not see it as clearly, he would know his condition was worsening.

To find a surgeon, he sought the help of his colleague and friend Danielle who had undergone multiple ocular surgeries. Given her past experiences, she "felt a particular connection to Brad's experience, that we shared a sense of private vulnerability." When looking for surgeon recommendations, she emphasized the importance of good communication skills and recognized the necessity of tailoring her approach to Brad's specific needs and desires.

"When I have accompanied people into a clinical encounter, tracking information and fielding questions has always been on the agenda, but beyond that everyone needed something different. My friend M needed me to transcribe her meetings with oncologists and then to laugh together about how her

---

66   Annie Robinson, Danielle Spencer, and Brad Lewis, "Illness Doula: Adding a New Role to Healthcare Practice," *Journal of Medical Humanities* 40, 2(2019):199-210.

67   Ibid.

doctor had such immaculately trimmed bangs...I would speak up if I felt there was critical information that would be important to make a decision; otherwise I was not to project any sort of agenda...my duty is clear: I am to be ego-less, in service to their needs, and responsive to what they might need in any given clinical encounter."[68]

This approach was crucial when Brad and his surgeon had trouble communicating which kind of lens correction to proceed with. While most elect for focuses on distance, he hoped for a close focus given his nearsightedness and the importance of reading and writing in his career. Given the surgeon could not understand why he would deviate from the norm, Danielle offered to attend the next appointment with him. Her presence in the room served to be a tremendous asset, as Brad now had someone with whom he could discuss certain interactions with medical professionals that seemed problematic and express his concerns.

As a mediator, Danielle helped by reframing certain questions and steering the conversation in a productive direction, recognizing her relative emotional detachment allowed her to approach the situation calmly and help Brad and his surgeon to understand each other. While it may not have seemed that way to Brad initially, the surgeon "seemed to genuinely care, to be invested in the encounter, and when we were able to break through this impasse, she seemed pleased and relieved, just as we were."[69]

---

68   Ibid.
69   Ibid.

In their article, Brad, Danielle, and their colleague Annie provide the narrative of Brad's experience while simultaneously advocating for an expansion of the doula role into different sectors of the medical field. Facilitating this transition would allow for an increased adoption of the practice of narrative medicine, through which providers can more deeply listen to their patient's needs, "not just with an ear for biological symptoms but with a heart for biographical stories and a keen sense of narrative understanding."[70] Having an extra person would alleviate stress for both patient and clinician alike, as they can serve as a further source of emotional support as well as a sounding board, intermediary, and/or advocate.

While I am a major proponent of the implementation of an "illness doula" or of the roles of social workers and patient advocates to help empower patients to take charge of their medical decisions, there are definitely challenges in the implementation of a doula-like role across the medical system, as highlighted by Leis, Spencer, and Robinson. In many cases, doulas are an out-of-pocket expense, with their services not covered (if so, only partially) by insurance, so access to this support is already limited to those who can afford it. While I am not saying those who can afford to hire a doula need their support less than those who cannot, there are many medical conditions that disproportionately affect certain marginalized populations, especially lower socioeconomic statuses, all of whom would benefit from having an advocate to help navigate them through the health care system and understand what services are available to them.

---

70   Ibid.

Aside from a financial standpoint, education also raises several concerns. While doulas do not receive any formal education, the process of becoming a certified doula ranges from several months to a year of education to gain a thorough understanding of the entire scope of pregnancy and practical experience with labor. With this in mind, it would be very difficult to establish a "universal doula" that had the same knowledge and proficiency in an array of fields. This models the common "jack of all trades, master of none" dilemma. Theoretically, doulas would either have to undergo specialized training in a field of their choice or receive a generalized training in understanding medical terminology and patient advocacy, with the former limiting the number of available doulas and the latter compromising their level of proficiency.

However, the most important concern with including illness doulas in current models of medical care is the difficulty in establishing a profound emotional connection with those whom they serve. Given the long duration of pregnancy and the potential for postpartum engagement, doulas have a substantial amount of time to get to know the mother and her family, understand their beliefs, and advocate for care that is in their best interests. While a similar approach would be beneficial for patients with chronic conditions or long-term treatments, it might not be as successful for short-term patients. In many cases, patients may receive the earth-shattering news of a surprising diagnosis and be forced to make monumental decisions about their care in very short time periods. While a doula or social worker equipped in medical lexicon may help the patient better understand the process, the same rapport and trust is very difficult to achieve in a such a short time span and may increase the risk of miscommunication and misunderstanding.

This brings up the primary question I had while considering the application of a universal doula: *how can we provide an advocate for short-term patients that is knowledgeable enough about their specific scenario without compromising the emotional aspects of the relationship?* Let's not forget while Brad's initial search criteria for a physician surely valued their expertise, his main focus was finding a health professional with a good bedside manner.

BEING THE BEST CHEERLEADER POSSIBLE: WHAT WE CAN LEARN FROM THE DOULA MINDSET

While being a patient in a hospital can be terrifying and difficult, watching your own loved ones undergo hospitalization or any kind of medical treatment is equally, if not more, terrifying and difficult. We are forced to watch our parents, siblings, cousins, elders, and even children suffer and at times it feels like all we can do is sit on the sidelines helplessly. It is one of the closest things to being in a real-life horror movie.

However, while it may seem silly or like it won't make much of a difference, perhaps the best advice I can give is the following: channel your inner Miami Heat dancer.

While I don't think any kind of gyrations or eight-beat performances may miraculously cure your loved ones from their illnesses (although laughter has been said to be one of the best forms of medicine), it is important you are able to maintain a strong and positive outlook, even during the bleakest of times. Although you may not have the same training or knowledge as a doula, you have had more time than any medical professional to develop a meaningful emotional connection with the patient and have already established a strong sense of their trust, making you a valuable part of this process. Based on the lessons I learned from conversations with doctors, patients, doulas, and Karen's knowledgeable teachers, here are some valuable tips I have gathered to be the best personal cheerleader for those you love:

BE THE BASE OF THE PYRAMID, NOT THE POINT.
While our widened and amazed eyes are usually drawn to the cheerleader smiling confidently at the top of any human pyramid, it is essential to remember she could not get up there nor get down without a strong and balanced community. Like that of a cheerleader, the support system for a patient contains many layers of strength and expertise, including nurses, surgeons, physicians, hospital staff, and, of course, their friends and family. And while their medical professionals may know more about how to treat their conditions, your loved ones heavily value your presence and affection. No one is asking you to make the discovery that cures their illness or to use the scalpel yourself: just hold their hand and be there for them every step of the way. Once they leave that hospital, you are the one who will get them through recovery and make sure they are capable of getting back on top of the pyramid again.

FOCUS ON THE FUNDAMENTALS.
Behind every routine filled with complex moves and acrobatics dancers perform effortlessly, there are hours and hours of practice that start with fundamentals. Before anyone can get

to the advanced steps, they must start from the beginning and work their way up. While no one expects you to know all the medical terminology surrounding your loved one's diagnosis or the mechanisms behind different treatment methods, it is important to become informed about the condition to engage in conversation with both the patient and their health professionals regarding treatment.

ALWAYS MAINTAIN GOOD SPORTSMANSHIP.

Regardless of whether things are going good or bad, it is important to cultivate an environment of respect between yourself, the patient, and all health professionals involved. While this experience will certainly be an emotional rollercoaster, approaching conflicts of interest firmly but professionally is essential because the only person that can get harmed is the patient. Remember you all are on the same team.

CONSIDER TRYING SOME NEW TRICKS.

While there are many common treatment modalities for specific procedures, it is always good to consider all potential options, even those that may seem somewhat unconventional. Although some may consider taking an epidural and delivering a baby in a hospital bed to be a standard approach to childbirth, many of Karen's instructors highlighted a myriad of approaches that can be enlisted, from bearing your child in the comfort of your own home, delivering them using a peanut ball in a birthing center, opting for a scheduled Cesarean section, or of course, conducting a water birth, perhaps even in your own kitchen. It is important to seek out the best healing process for your loved one, even if that means daring to be different and taking a risk.

BE THEIR BIGGEST FAN!

At the end of the day, the most important thing to remember is you are building these skills to best support your loved ones in any way you can. For some, you may need to push them to voice their questions or make them adhere to their treatment protocol if they are stubborn or forgetful. Other patients may be confident enough to be vocal and just need you there to cheer them on and hold their hand. While this process can be emotionally challenging and it can be easy for both of you to get overwhelmed by your feelings, do your best to stay strong and act in the best interests of the patient. Maybe you both need a good cry to get all the feelings out or some inappropriately timed jokes to remember there's so much more to life than being in a medical setting. There's no one right answer here.

Lastly, make sure they know regardless of what the score ends up being, you'll always cheer them on every step of the way and in the wake of the next challenge, they can count on you to be the base of their pyramid.

CHAPTER 10

IMPORTANT TOOLS FOR HEALTH PROFESSIONALS

———

As her day at work begins, Dr. Miranda Bailey is paged by Dr. Richard Webber, Chief of Surgery, to meet her on the roof. She walks up to the helipad, confused as to why nothing is there. Upon finding Dr. Webber, he proceeds to praise her for conducting an effective domino surgery the previous week, during which she performed six successive kidney transplants. Impressed by her performance, he now comes to her with a special task: she needs to form a team of surgeons to save a ten-year-old girl with an inoperable tumor.[71]

Dr. Bailey is initially taken aback by the challenge but knows she must do everything to provide this girl with the chance to live a happy and healthy life. She marches confidently to

---

71 *Grey's Anatomy*, season 5, episode 6, "Life During Wartime," directed by James Frawley, written by Mark Wilding, featuring Ellen Pompeo, Sandra Oh, and Katherine Heigl, aired October 30, 2008, on ABC.

the resident locker room where she must select a resident to join her team.[72]

When informing her residents they will get to skip the mandatory skills lab to operate on this young girl, Cristina, Alex, George, and Izzie all eagerly raise their hands and try to prove themselves worthy of joining the surgery. However, Dr. Bailey is instead drawn to Meredith, who holds her childhood doll she recently found.[73]

Intrigued, Dr. Bailey asks "Grey, is that Anatomy Jane?"[74]

"Yes," she responds, with a somewhat perplexed expression on her face as she looks down at the plastic, brunette-haired doll adorned with bright blue scrubs.[75]

"With the twenty-four removable organs and the optional parts to simulate pregnancy?"[76]

"Yes. Does that mean I'm out too?"[77]

"No, that means you're in," Dr. Bailey says, much to the surprise of Dr. Grey and her peers.[78]

---

72   Ibid.
73   Ibid.
74   Ibid.
75   Ibid.
76   Ibid.
77   Ibid.
78   Ibid.

A few scenes later, we see Dr. Bailey and her team meeting with the young girl and her family to discuss her diagnosis. Dr. Grey begins with an overview of the patient's condition:

"Tori Begler, age ten. Tori has an abdominal leiomyosarcoma. The tumor is wrapped around her celiac artery, her splenic artery, and her left gastric artery. It is considered unresectable."[79]

As one might predict, Tori looks overwhelmed by the complex information that just left Dr. Grey's mouth. Her family members fondly look at their daughter with confusion and concern, as Tori stares blankly at Dr. Bailey.[80]

Dr. Bailey smiles and asks, "Did you understand a word of that Tori?"[81]

"Not really," she says, as the two of them nervously chuckle.[82]

Dr. Grey proceeds to try explaining again, this time with the help of Anatomy Jane. "This is Anatomy Jane."[83]

"She's kind of funny looking," Tori quips with a smile on her face.[84]

---

79   Ibid.
80   Ibid.
81   Ibid.
82   Ibid.
83   Ibid.
84   Ibid.

"She is funny looking, but she's very helpful. The tumor is way down here in your belly," Dr. Grey explains as she removes the skin flap protecting Anatomy Jane's organs and points to her stomach.[85] "It's hard to get at because it's underneath all these organs." Tori and her family members watch as Dr. Grey references the locations of the tumor, nodding and now appearing to understand and even feel slightly relieved.[86]

While Shonda Rhimes' hit television show *Grey's Anatomy* is primarily known for its dramatic storylines and (mc) steamy romances, this scene provides an important example that displays the power of patient education in preoperative care. Although the team of medical professionals did not provide an immediate solution for the resection of Tori's tumor, the simple act of explaining the nature of the tumor in comprehensible terms, rather than using complex medical jargon, better prepared Tori and her family to approach a conversation about her treatment plan without feeling overwhelmed. Simultaneously, the use of a simple visual aid like Anatomy Jane helped them visualize the otherwise invisible threat to Tori's health, making it a little less scary to deal with.

Although I have not had any experience as a health professional, the process of writing this book and hearing people's stories has provided me with a unique opportunity to learn from individuals who have experienced all facets of the field, from patients living through it to physicians trying to change it from within. By sharing some of their stories and

---

85   Ibid.
86   Ibid.

experiences, I hope to provide some insight to those seeking to work in health professions as to how they can best use their roles to empower patients to advocate for themselves and taste THEIR OWN medicine.

UNDERSTANDING YOUR TARGET AUDIENCE

Having gone through an extensive and rigorous education that required the memorization of a myriad of biochemical mechanisms and anatomical terms, it is not surprising people working in health-related careers often sound like they are speaking another language. However, while this language may be necessary when speaking with their peers to discuss the mechanics of an upcoming surgery or determining a diagnosis, it is not usually received well by patients and their families, most of whom lack a similar proficiency in medical terminology.

A case report written by Bell and Condren (2016) provides some important communication strategies specifically tailored to empower child patients. In a pediatric setting, age plays a major role in the degree to which a patient is involved in their medical care, with parents taking the lead until their child can fully process information about their health. While Bell and Condren provide some amazing strategies on establishing rapport with child patients and their families, I was especially intrigued by a figure they included that applies Jean Piaget's theory and stages of cognitive development to teaching a child about the use of amoxicillin to treat ear infections.[87]

---

87   Jennifer Bell and Michelle Condren, "Communication Strategies for Empowering and Protecting Children," *The Journal of Pediatric Pharmacology and Therapeutics* 21, 2(2016):176-184.

In the figure, they provide a range of responses that increase in complexity as the child matures and their ability to comprehend information improves. For example, when explaining the importance of continuing to take antibiotic medication to prevent bacteria from developing resistance, a physician may tell a child between seven and eleven years of age "It's important to take it every day for ten days so your infection doesn't come back."[88] However, a child who has passed the age of twelve and whose logical reasoning skills better equip them to understand and control their illness may instead be told, "You should start feeling better in two days, but it is important to keep taking it even if you start feeling better so the infection doesn't come back."[89]

While these assumptions may vary from case to case based on the child's previous exposure to health settings or level of comprehension in general, Bell and Condren provide valuable insight on how to effectively engage the child in the conversation, rather than solely talking to their caregivers. I especially appreciated that between the Concrete Operations and Formal Operations stages, the final question changes from "**Do** you have any questions for me?" to "**What** questions do you have for me?"[90] By framing questions in an open-ended manner that does not elicit a yes-or-no response, medical professionals empower the child to become active in the conversation about their health, even if just to say they have nothing to ask.

---

88 Ibid.
89 Ibid.
90 Ibid.

At the same time, it is important to create an atmosphere in which children are comfortable sharing these questions and directly conversing with their health professionals rather than deflecting immediately to their caregivers (assuming they have reached the appropriate adolescent age, of course). I had the amazing opportunity to discuss such approaches with Dr. Igor Shumskiy, a pediatric specialist and chief medical officer of Nurse-1-1, a HIPAA-compliant service that provides patients with quick and personalized correspondence with a nurse who can help them navigate their health-related circumstances directly from their mobile devices. Dr. Igor always provides adolescents the opportunity to speak with him independently of their parents by asking the caregiver(s) to briefly exit the room. This allows the adolescent to speak more comfortably about potential sensitive topics, such as sexual health or substance use, which the adolescent may not be as transparent about in the presence of their caregiver. He likes to remind the patient "I am your doctor, not your parents' doctor" and everything they discuss is confidential, unless the adolescent is having suicidal or homicidal thoughts.

Additionally, he ensures his patients they will not be judged or criticized based on what their answers are to his questions. Regardless of the patient's level of sexual activity, sexual preference, gender identity, race, or socioeconomic status, he tries to foster an environment where the adolescent feels safe and supported, an essential atmosphere for patients regardless of what age they are. If patients are curious about learning more about their conditions and what they can do to maintain a healthy lifestyle, he also makes an effort to send them papers and research articles they can comprehend based on their level of literacy to feed their curiosity and keep them engaged. During our conversation, Dr. Igor simultaneously emphasized cultivating a similar rapport and trust with a patient's loved ones, especially parents, as they are essential support systems in the process of recovery. Many times, he has found parents will frequently dance around a specific issue with their child that worries them, such as a persistent cold or feelings of weakness and fatigue, but they may not admit what's actually worrying them, fearful of being embarrassed for using Google for medical advice. Dr. Igor acknowledged the important role of a provider to affirm patients and caregivers alike that there are no stupid questions and stated while there may be a knowledge imbalance, there should NOT be a power imbalance when it comes to communication and decision-making. By directly asking them "What are you really worried about?" a health professional welcomes individuals to speak their truth and can provide them with the valuable assurance that will encourage and allow them to continue being active and engaged in conversation and the treatment process as a whole.

As a former child and adolescent patient, I especially appreciated when my doctors took the time to address me directly regarding any concerns and questions I had, although my interest was usually directed toward how the machine determining the prescription for my new glasses worked or why the jelly they put on my abdomen for my yearly kidney ultrasound was so warm. Nonetheless, it is essential health information is provided in a clear and comprehensible fashion, especially for younger patients, so they can be actively engaged in conversations and empowered to make informed decisions about their well-being.

EMBRACING CREATIVE MEDIUMS

While effective and transparent verbal communication between health professionals and those whom they serve is a cornerstone of patient-centered care, it is important to remember each patient is unique and has different needs based on their lived experiences, described by the National Clinical Guideline Centre as follows:

"The recognition that individuals are living with their condition and experiencing it in a unique way, that family and broader life need to be taken into account, and that all of these aspects of lived experience can affect self-care. Taking into account individual physical needs and cognitive needs because of condition. Everyday experiences, hopes, expectations, future uncertainty, feelings of loss, feelings of being morally judged, feelings of blame. Some of these experiences originate 'outside' of the health care system but are brought with the patient into the health system; other experiences may be affected by attitudes and expectations of health professionals."[91]

Although a patient's symptoms may be "textbook" for a specific condition, all facets of their lifestyle and identity need to be considered when curating the best treatment plan and even when communicating with them. I had an interesting discussion about personalized care with my friend Olivia at Vanderbilt. During our chat, we both shared our respective exposures in health care settings. As a high school student, Olivia was diagnosed with cancer, which caused some very tremendous

---

91   National Clinician Guideline Centre (UK). *Patient Experience in Adult NHS Services: Improving the Experience of Care for People Using Adult NHS Services: Patient Experience in Generic Terms* (London: Royal College of Physicians (UK), 2012).

lifestyle shifts. Having been used to taking many advanced classes coupled with being involved in different clubs and organizations, she found it difficult to suddenly decrease her course load and let go of many of her commitments. In many ways, the experience of being a patient made her lose sight of her own identity as a person before her illness and she wished more of her health professionals took the time to talk to her about this and see what she needed in those moments.

Touched by the nurses who took the time to talk to her about her feelings and needs throughout the treatment process, Olivia volunteers with the Child Life Specialists at the Vanderbilt University Medical Center. When interacting with child patients, her main goal is to provide them with what they need in that exact moment, whether it be playing a game with them, sitting in silence, or providing a listening ear to vent to. Through this role, she hopes to provide these children with the support and love necessary so they don't lose sight of who they are because while they may be a patient in the hospital, they are human beings above all.

These acknowledgments and considerations are key for medical professionals to consider to provide impactful patient-centered care and can especially be applied to communication with patients about their diagnoses, symptoms, and treatments. Just as teachers combine lectures with audiovisual components and analogies to appeal to the different learning styles of all of their students, a similar approach in educating patients can be just as, if not more, valuable.

For example, the use of analogies in health care is an effective technique in facilitating effective community between health professionals and patients. As stated by Anatole Broyard in his autobiography *Intoxicated by my Illness and Other Writings on Life and Death*, "Metaphors may be as necessary to illness as they are to literature, as comforting to the patient as his own bathrobe and slippers. At the very least, they are a relief from medical terminology... Perhaps only metaphor can express the bafflement, the panic combined with beatitude, of the threatened person."[92]

The use of metaphors in medicine has been shown to be extremely valuable in introducing unfamiliar information to patients and their families in a comprehensible manner, while also dispelling misconceptions counterproductive to the healing process.[93] The use of war metaphors that paint the patient as a soldier in combat at the line of fire can help motivate patients to fight their illness to the end, whereas sports metaphors place patients, caregivers, and their providers on the same team as they work together to achieve victory over their shared opponent: the illness. By facilitating these mindsets and personalizing metaphors to the unique interests of patients, health professionals can both strengthen the doctor-patient relationship and improve their patients' resilience and motivation as they face adversity head on.

As seen through Dr. Grey's use of Anatomy Jane, it is also beneficial to incorporate audiovisual components into explanations of health-related concepts, especially given the alarming statistics surrounding health literacy and the general complexity of medical terminology. Brian Rodvien, the

---

92 Vyjeyanthi S Periyakoil, "Using Metaphors in Medicine," *The Journal of Palliative Medicine* 11, 6(2008):842-844.

93 Ibid.

CEO and founder of Smarter Medical Care, is one such individual who has dedicated his work to building these types of patient resources. Smarter Medical Care is a company that produces patient education videos on various health topics, such as detailing specific illnesses or describing certain procedures, to help navigate the confusion and anxiety that often surrounds a patient's diagnosis.

As Brian explained to me during a conversation we had last summer, "If we can give the right information to the patient and their family at the right time, we can reduce their anxiety. This will heighten the likelihood that they will have a more productive conversation with their healthcare professionals resulting in a better quality of life."

During a normal year, Smarter Medical Care produces about one hundred patient education videos in a variety of languages, including English, Spanish, French, German, Italian, and Russian, that allow patients of varying literacy levels to better understand certain facets of the treatment process. The medium of animation has been shown to "improve participants' ability to identify personal information-gaps, engage in meaningful community-level dialogue, and ask questions about health research," especially given its nonthreatening and lively nature is very beneficial in promoting the recall of information. Animations are easily translated to account for different cultural and linguistic barriers that may hinder one's understanding of key health information.[94] Learning

---

94   Shiba George, Erin Moran, Nelida Duran, and Robert A. Jenders, "Using Animation as an Information Tool to Advance Health Research Literacy among Minority Participants," *AMIA Annual Symposium Procurement*, (2013):475-84.

from his experiences as a patient, a family member to his mother who passed away from cancer, and his father's experiences as a successful physician, Brian hopes to provide medical information in a unique and palatable manner that will better engage and empower patients in their own care.

By embracing creative approaches such as those aforementioned, medical professionals can further enhance the quality of communication they have with their patients and facilitate patients' greater understanding of their own health and well-being. Rather than seeking a "one size fits all" approach to treatment, it is important to push the boundaries and try new methods to ensure each individual is given and receives the best care possible.

SELF-CARE AND THE THREATS OF COMPASSION FATIGUE AND PHYSICIAN BURNOUT

"Numerous global studies involving nearly every medical and surgical specialty indicate that approximately one of every three physicians is experiencing burnout at any given time."[95]

As patients and loved ones of patients, we look up to health professionals, seeing them as heroes, magicians, and saviors doing the work of a higher power. However, at times

---

95   Dike Drummond, "Part I: Burnout Basics – Symptoms, Effects, Prevalence and the Five Main Causes," *Missouri Medicine* 113, 4(2016):252-255.

this idolization makes it especially hard for both us and health professionals alike to see them for what they truly are behind their scrubs or white coats: human beings. While health professionals are admired and respected, living up to this expectation can be extremely exhausting and have serious impacts on providers' mental, physical, and emotional health.

While statistics surrounding leading causes of death in the United States, such as cardiovascular disease, cancer, diabetes, and suicide, are at the forefront of the press, attention should also be drawn to the alarming rates of physician burnout and compassion fatigue directly harming the individuals who fight to protect us from these threats. In 2020 alone, 42 percent of physicians reported they felt burned out due to factors such as long work hours, extensive bureaucratic tasks (e.g. paperwork and charting), and a lack of support.[96]

Dr. Anthony Orsini, a neonatologist and founder of The Orsini Way, discusses these very real issues in an episode of *Difficult Conversations: Lessons I Learned as an ICU Physician*, which provides communication training programs used at medical schools and residency programs across the country based on Dr. Orsini's extensive research and experience both as a physician and a child with chronic illness. In this particular episode, he interviewed Dr. Dike Drummond, a Mayo Clinic trained family doctor, professional coach, author,

---

96   Leslie Kane, "Medscape National Physician Burnout & Suicide Report 2020: The Generational Divide," Medscape, last modified January 15, 2020.

speaker, and trainer focused on tackling the "modern epidemic of professional burnout."[97]

Dr. Drummond explains every health care professional, regardless of their position, walks into a small whirlwind whenever they enter the workplace. "Things are coming at you from all different directions. Patients only bring complaints. Your staff only bring prompts, questions, decisions, responsibility, busy work, charting, all that kind of stuff. It's like being in a whirlwind...from the inside... all you could see is the inside walls...and most of what you see sucks. So the question is, how do you step out of your whirlwind?"[98] What makes escaping this whirlwind especially difficult stems from the rigorous education programs providers are put through, which, according to Dr. Drummond, program them to see things like fatigue, hunger, and even using the bathroom as signs of weakness that must be hidden from their peers and colleagues. However, internalizing these sources of distress and fatigue only diminishes the performance of such individuals, and, in effect, compromises the quality of care given to patients, which nobody wants.[99]

Both Dr. Drummond and Dr. Orsini provide valuable examples of methods to mitigate such burnout and fatigue. For example, Dr. Drummond's "SqueeGee Breath" technique involves taking a deep breath from the nose or mouth,

---

97   Anthony Orsini, "Difficult Conversations About Physician Burnout with Dr. Dike Drummond," September 21, 2020, in *Difficult Conversations – Lessons I Learned as an ICU Physician with Dr. Anthony Orsini,* podcast, MP3 audio, 40:34.
98   Ibid.
99   Ibid.

holding it in for two to three seconds, releasing the breath through one's toes for two to three seconds, all the while imagining a giant squeegee has completely wiped away your problems and sources of distress. Additionally, he emphasizes the importance of focusing on small goals and actions you can perform now to increase the level of overlap between the values and organization of your current practice and the ideal perception of medicine you may have formed as early as when you decided to go to medical school.[100]

Dr. Orsini provides similar strategies and discusses their implementation in his *It's All in the Delivery* program, which aims to improve patient experience and satisfaction by training medical staff on how to communicate and connect with other human beings. He emphasizes the value of having even small conversations with patients about unrelated topics to their health, such as current sports events, connecting with them beyond the information on their chart, and holding health professionals at levels of expertise accountable to ensure no one becomes trapped in the whirlwind.[101]

As stated by Professor Teresa Hellín of Alcalá University, "To attend those who suffer, a physician must possess not only the scientific knowledge and technical abilities, but also an understanding of human nature. The patient is not just a group of symptoms, damaged organs and altered emotions. The patient is a human being, at the same time worried and hopeful, who is searching for relief, help and trust. The importance of an intimate relationship between patient and

---

100 Ibid.
101 Ibid.

physician can never be overstated because in most cases an accurate diagnosis, as well as an effective treatment, relies directly on the quality of this relationship."[102]

Given the unique and immense value of the relationship between a patient and their health care professional, it is essential both parties put in the necessary effort to develop a strong rapport that will guide all approaches and morale throughout the treatment process. However, since patients seek the expertise and guidance of physicians to guide their own care, it is important medical professionals ensure their own physical and emotional health are optimal so they can put their best foot forward for those whom they serve.

I had the unique opportunity of attending a virtual guest lecture given by Dr. David Langer, the chairman of the department of neurosurgery at Lennox Hill Hospital in New York City. If any of this sounds familiar, that's because his life, among those of three other medical professionals practicing at the facility, was explored through the popular documentary web television series on Netflix called *Lennox Hill*, which premiered during the summer of 2020. While he provided a lot of valuable insight regarding how to approach challenges both as premedical students and as human beings in general, I especially appreciated his commentary on how he copes with physician burnout, something that has especially been exacerbated by the COVID-19 pandemic. According to a survey by Medscape completed by over 7,500 physicians worldwide, almost five thousand of which practice

---

102 R. Kaba and P. Sooriakumaran, "The Evolution of the Doctor-Patient Relationship," *International Journal of Surgery* 5, 1(2007):57-65.

medicine in the United States, 64 percent of US physicians reported their sense of burnout had been intensified by the pandemic, with 29 percent reporting increased eating, 19 percent reporting increased drinking of alcohol, and 2 percent reporting increased usage of prescription stimulants and medications.[103]

As a practicing physician with a lot of experience, Dr. Langer admitted to us he did indeed experience burnout at times, especially given the current global climate. He explained that given the hectic nature of the job, it is common for health professionals to compact their emotions to keep pushing, but also emphasized the importance of giving oneself the opportunity to take a break. Putting forth your best effort is all you can do and no matter how much you improve in your career, you are still susceptible of experiencing failure. However, the most important thing is not the failure itself, but how one responds to it. Rather than ignoring your mistakes and shortcomings or letting them define you, Dr. Langer expressed the importance of learning from these experiences and using them to make yourself better, advice that is relevant to both physician burnout and essentially every career out there. It is important in times of hardship, we lean on those we love, adapt to changes, and approach problems with creativity and open-mindedness because if you don't get what you want, it is ultimately up to you to make your desires a reality.

Remember as a health professional, you can only help others be at their best if you are at your best. Self-care looks different

---

103   Leslie Kane, "Medscape."

for everyone, much like treatment plans, so when you write your next prescription of medications and behaviors necessary for your patient, don't forget to prescribe yourself the ingredients you need to prepare the best recipe for your own wellness.

CONCLUSION

Some of you might be thinking, "Well this was cool, but I won't be seeing my primary care physician for another year." Others might be knee-deep in a treatment plan and feel they're too far into the process to begin engaging in such advocacy. And the pessimists (who I have hopefully since converted) might claim the health care industry isn't changing anytime soon, so there is no point in changing anything.

So where do we go from here?

Let me remind you being a curious patient does not begin the second you put on that gown and hop into that hospital bed. It begins now, when you put down this book and decide whether you're going to nap on the couch for the next hour (like I most probably will after finishing up this conclusion) or go for an eight-mile run (like my roommate who is currently tying his shoelaces while I sit across from him in my pajamas).

Our health and well-being isn't defined by the big decisions we make when faced with life-or-death circumstances; it is constantly shaped by the choices we make in our everyday lives, whether it be our diet, lifestyle, or attitudes. Before we can learn how to advocate for ourselves in health care settings, we need to begin empowering ourselves every day to maintain our health and well-being.

In Part one, I introduced you to some foundational knowledge surrounding the history of the doctor-patient relationship and health education in the United States and explored how the ideas of autonomy and intrinsic motivation influence the choices we make. That being said, the overview I provided was very general and I would highly recommend further exploring these topics to best prepare yourself for your given situation or if you're just interested in learning more about the different dimensions of health care delivery.

In Part two, we dissected the idea of the curious patient through my personal experiences with the health care system and the best ways in which they can be supported by their caregivers through my insightful journey as an "expecting mother." During these chapters, I emphasized the importance of being strong and confident as you engage in conversation with your health professionals, but I'd also like to remind you again to not disregard the importance of self-care. Your emotional state is extremely impactful on your physical and mental well-being and recognizing what you're feeling will only enhance the quality of your relationship with your providers and the care you ultimately receive.

In Part three, I provided actionable steps you can start implementing right away in health care settings, whether it be as a patient, a loved one, or even a medical professional. The nature of health care delivery is one that is constantly evolving, which is especially visible now, and it is important we are flexible and resilient as we adapt to the changes. However, it is just as, if not more crucial we do not sacrifice our own well-being as we navigate these changes. By using our resources responsibly and effectively and treating each other with empathy and compassion, we can ensure the genuine human connection between patient and provider is not lost in the cracks.

As you navigate current and future health experiences, remember you know your body best and you have a say in making the final decision. If you feel uncomfortable with a certain course of treatment or prefer to explore another alternative, articulate that to your health care provider and start a conversation with them to explore what option will truly cater to your best interests.

However, also keep in mind this approach goes beyond medical settings and should be implemented into your daily lifestyle. While I may have bashed naps earlier (I promise I am a big nap proponent), it takes a lot of strength to recognize your limits and to acknowledge when your body needs rest. At the same time, I would also encourage you to keep an open mind and dare to venture out of your comfort zone when it's in your best interests. As a water sport athlete, I found myself gasping for air and screaming internally after my roommate miraculously convinced me to join him on an eight-mile run, but I finished it with a clear mind, a positive spirit, and less guilt during my midnight spoonful of Nutella. At the end of the day, it's all about balance.

When I first introduced you to the stories I've shared throughout this book, I asked you to listen. Now that you've listened enough, it's time to let yourself be heard.

Trust in the power of your voice, in your awareness of your body, and in the capabilities of your health care providers.

Be the best advocate for yourself and for your loved ones in these situations and in your capacity for empathy and resilience.

Recognize that regardless of your strength and your education, these situations can be emotionally overwhelming and it's okay to ask for help. Your health care providers want to help you and your loved ones and if you ignore your feelings, you won't be able to put your best foot forward.

With the research, narratives, and actionable advice I have outlined throughout this book, I really hope, and I mean this with the utmost sincerity, you can finally get a taste of YOUR OWN medicine.

ACKNOWLEDGMENTS

To my incredible family and amazing friends, thank you so much for the lessons I've learned, the love I've received, and the memories I'll always cherish. I couldn't ask for a more incredible group of people to carry throughout my life.

Mom, thank you for always supporting all of my endeavors, even when it's clear I should've stopped boiling the ramen five minutes ago.

Dad, thank you for always reminding me to take things easy. I truly am proud to be your son.

But most of all,

Sophie, Lucy, and Lily, thank you so much for your unwavering moral support. Your constant tendencies to take naps on my computer and incessant barking for belly rubs was an instrumental and appreciated part of the creative process I will never forget.

Thank you to all of my incredible mentors throughout my life for your guidance, especially my science teachers. While a lot of glassware broke in the process, I'm grateful your faith in me never did.

Thank you to all of my incredible interviewees who took time out of their busy schedules to share the insights and stories that filled the spaces between my corny attempts at humor. In a particularly isolating time for the world, I truly appreciate your willingness to connect and I hope our paths cross again.

Thank you so much to all the incredible people I had the opportunity to work with via the Creator Institute. To my fellow authors, I could not have asked for a more supportive and talented cohort and I cannot wait to see the incredible things you all continue to do. To my beta readers, thank you for taking the time to read my preliminary drafts and for providing your feedback. Lastly, thank you so much to everyone who has influenced my creative process and inspired my stories, especially Eric Koester, Diedre Hammons, Brian Bies, Lisa Patterson, Ruslan Nabiev, and Amanda Moskowitz.

Thank you so much to everyone who preordered a copy of the book or donated to my presale campaign. I am immensely grateful you all decided to support me along this journey and, as promised, you are in the book (listed in alphabetical order).

Abraham Awad

Brian Stoffers

Ajay Dungar

Elizabeth Perez

Anil Idnani

Eric Koester

Antonia Lemann

Frances Batista

Bobby Singh

Geetu Mirpuri

Gregory Nguyen
Harry Chandi
Justin Holmes
Kingsley Firth
Kishin Mirpuri
Kumar Mukhi
Maristella Cartafina
Mattigan Kelly
Michael Gonçalves
Natasha Kaycee
Neel Tripuraneni
Pamela Nielsen
Peter Papangelis
R. Swidorowicz
Rafael Gill
Raj Amit Mirpuri

Rajesh Mirpuri
Ralph Quintero
Regan Dumas
Sabrina Mirpuri
Sanguita Chandi
Sanjay Dhingreja
Sheline Chandi
Simran Khiantani
Sunaina Mirchandani
Sunya Chandi
Thierry Chaunu
Timothy F Gearty
Tyler Mittelman
Yoly McCarthy
Zeinab Ramos

Last but not least, thank you to Joseph Sexton for sending me the Google Form link one fateful summer day that caused this journey to happen in the first place. I truly cherish our friendship and hope we can continue to be there for each other in the important moments.

If your name is not here, know that I love and appreciate you for the influence you've had on my life, positive or negative. If not for you, I wouldn't be here, and for that I am very grateful.

APPENDIX

———

INTRODUCTION

Center for Health Care Strategies. "What is Health Literacy?". 2013. https://www.chcs.org/media/What_is_Health_Literacy.pdf.

Fadiman, Anne. *The Spirit Catches You and You Fall Down: A Hmong Child, Her American Doctors, and the Collision of Two Cultures.* New York: Farrar, Straus and Giroux, 1997.

TEDx Talks. "Advocate for Your Health | Molly Hottle | TEDxTucson." March 6, 2017. Video, 14:56. https://www.youtube.com/watch?v=Grs5r-Soq5nk.

CHAPTER 1

Harrison, Natalie. "Regressing or progressing: what next for the doctor–patient relationship?." *The Lancet* 6, 3(2018):178-180. https://doi.org/10.1016/S2213-2600(18)30075-4.

Johnson, Tyler. "The Importance of Physician-Patient Relationships Communication and Trust in Health Care." Duke Center for Personalized Health Care. Last modified March 11, 2019. https://dukepersonalizedhealth.org/2019/03/the-importance-of-physician-patient-relationships-communication-and-trust-in-health-care/.

Luciano, Michael C. "The Art of the Doctor-Patient Relationship in the COVID-19 Era." MEDPAGE TODAY. Last modified April 23, 2020. https://www.medpagetoday.com/infectiousdisease/covid19/86120.

Stanford Alumni. "The Doctor-Patient Relationship with Abraham Verghese." October 3, 2013. Video, 13:58. https://www.youtube.com/watch?v=VNrWb9w6JWE

CHAPTER 2

Anfinrund, Philip, Valentyn Stadnytskui, Christina E Bax, and Adriaan Bax. "Visualizing Speech-Generated Oral Fluid Droplets with Laser Light Scattering." *The New England Journal of Medicine* 382, 21(2020):2061-2063. https://doi.org/10.1056/NEJMc2007800.

Bai, Nina. "Still Confused About Masks? Here's the Science Behind How Face Masks Prevent Coronavirus." UCSF. Last modified July 11, 2020. https://www.ucsf.edu/news/2020/06/417906/still-confused-about-masks-heres-science-behind-how-face-masks-prevent.

Kounios, John and Mark Beeman. "How Incentives Hinder Innovation." *Behavioral Scientist.* September 03, 2015. https://behavioralscientist.org/how-incentives-hinder-innovation-creativity/.

Mayo Clinic. "Patient Experience with Shared Decision Making at Mayo Clinic." December 28, 2010. Video, 3:37. https://www.youtube.com/watch?v=QR3ODoSJQ38.

Wong, Brittany. "The Psychology Behind Why Some People Refuse To Wear Face Masks." *HuffPost.* July 01, 2020. https://www.huffpost.com/entry/psychology-why-people-refuse-wear-face-masks_l_5efb723cc5b-6ca970915bc53.

CHAPTER 3

Allensworth, Diane, Elaine Lawson, Lois Nicholson, and James Wyche, eds. *Schools and Health: Our Nation's Investment.* Washington DC: National Academies Press, 1997.

Center for Disease Control and Prevention. "Female Genital Cutting." Accessed October 29, 2020. https://www.cdc.gov/immigrantrefugeehealth/guidelines/domestic/general/discussion/female-genital-cutting.html.

Gigerenzer, Gerd, Wolfgang Gaissmaier, Elke Kurz-Milcke, Lisa M Schwartz, and Steven Woloshin. "Helping Doctors and Patients Make Sense of Health Statistics." *Psychological Science in the Public Interest* 8. 2(2007):53-96. https://www.doi.org/10.1111/j.1539-6053.2008.00033.x.

Harvard Health. "Navigating Health Insurance." Accessed December 26, 2020. https://www.health.harvard.edu/staying-healthy/navigating-health-insurance.

McCarthy, Jennifer. "The Complete Guide to Health Insurance." The Simple Dollar. Last modified August 28, 2020. https://www.thesimpledollar.com/financial-wellness/health-insurance-guide.

Pieri, Sophie. "Navigating Health Insurance." Global Genes. Last modified February 09, 2021. https://globalgenes.happyfox.com/kb/article/26-navigating-health-insurance/.

Videto, Donna M. and Joseph A. Drake. "Promoting Health Literacy Through Defining and Measuring Quality School Health Education"." *Health Promotion Practice* 20, 6(2019):824-833. https://doi.org/10.1177/1524839919870194.

CHAPTER 4

Garfinkel, Sarah N., Emma Zorab, Nakulan Navaratnam, Miriam Engels, Núria Mallorquí-Bagué, Ludovico Minati, Nicholas G Dowell, Jos F. Brosschot, Julian F. Thayer, and Hugo D. Critchley. "Anger in brain and body: the neural and physiological perturbation of decision-making by emotion." *Social Cognitive and Affective Neuroscience* 11, 1(2016):150-8. https://doi.org/10.1093/scan/nsv099.

Johns Hopkins Medicine. "Dealing With Difficult Emotions." Accessed October 29, 2020. https://www.hopkinsallchildrens.org/Patients-Families/Health-Library/HealthDocNew/Dealing-With-Difficult-Emotions.

Kusev, Petko, Harry Purser, Renata Heilman, Alex J. Cooke, Paul Van Shaik, Victoria Baranova, Rose Martin, and Peter Ayton. "Understanding Risky Behavior: The Influence of Cognitive, Emotional and Hormonal Factors on Decision-Making under Risk." *Frontiers in Psychology 8*, 102(2017). https://doi.org/10.3389/fpsyg.2017.00102.

Kozlowski, Desirée, Marie Hutchinson, John Hurley, Joanne Rowley, and Joanna Sutherland. "The role of emotion in clinical decision making: an integrative literature review." *BMC Medical Education* 17, 255(2017). https://doi.org/10.1186/s12909-017-1089-7.

TEDx Talks. "TEDxMaastricht - Fred Lee - 'Patient Satisfaction or Patient Experience?.'" April 6, 2011. Video. 17:18. https://www.youtube.com/watch?v=tylvc9dY4o0

CHAPTER 5

DONA International. "What Is a Doula?" Accessed September 07, 2020. https://www.dona.org/what-is-a-doula/.

TEDx Talks. "What the Right Support Can Do For You: A Doula is More Than a Good Friend | Lin Liang | TEDxCUNY." May 14, 2019. Video, 12:51. https://www.youtube.com/watch?v=4c45U7tGqV8.

CHAPTER 7

How to Adult. "How to Choose a Doctor (in the U.S.)." September 13, 2017. Video, 4:27. https://www.youtube.com/watch?v=5Vi-PL1HPb8.

TEDx Talks. "Emily Ross: Life or Death: The Power of Health Advocacy." June 3, 2016. Video. 16:29. https://www.youtube.com/watch?v=5Z5k1i1vFxo.

CHAPTER 8

Coach Simona. "Episode 41: Obsessed with Googling Symptoms? Meet Cyberchondria." March 19, 2019. In *Simplify Your Life.* Podcast, MP3 Audio, 06:42. https://coachsimona.com/podcast/ep41-obsessed-googling-symptoms/.

Doctor.com. "2018 Customer experience trends in healthcare." Accessed on February 05, 2021. https://www.doctor.com/cxtrends2018.

Hill, Michella G., Moira Sim, and Brennen Mills. "The quality of diagnosis and triage advice provided by free online symptom checkers and apps in Australia." *The Medical Journal of Australia* 212, 11(2020):514-519. https://doi.org/10.5694/mja2.50600

Starcevic, Vladan, David Berle, and Sandra Arnáez. "Recent Insights Into Cyberchondria." *Current Psychiatry Reports* 22, 11(2020):56. https://doi.org/10.1007/s11920-020-01179-8

CHAPTER 9

Robinson, Annie, Danielle Spencer, and Brad Lewis. "Illness Doula: Adding a New Role to Healthcare Practice." *Journal of Medical Humanities* 40, 2(2019):199-210. https://doi.org/10.1007/s10912-017-9438-4

CHAPTER 10

Bell, Jennifer and Michelle Condren. "Communication Strategies for Empowering and Protecting Children." *The Journal of Pediatric Pharmacology and Therapeutics* 21, 2(2016):176-184. https://doi.org/10.5863/1551-6776-21.2.176

Drummond, Dike. "Part I: Burnout Basics – Symptoms, Effects, Prevalence and the Five Main Causes." *Missouri Medicine* 113, 4(2016):252-255. https://www.ncbi.nlm.nih.gov/pmc/articles/PMC6139917/

George, Shiba, Erin Moran, Nelida Duran, and Robert A. Jenders. "Using Animation as an Information Tool to Advance Health Research Literacy among Minority Participants." *AMIA Annual Symposium Procurement*, (2013):475-84. https://pubmed.ncbi.nlm.nih.gov/24551351/

Kaba, R. and P. Sooriakumaran, "The Evolution of the Doctor-Patient Relationship." *International Journal of Surgery* 5, 1(2007):57-65. https://doi.org/10.1016/j.ijsu.2006.01.005

Kane, Leslie. "Medscape National Physician Burnout & Suicide Report 2020: The Generational Divide." Medscape. Last modified January 15, 2020. https://www.medscape.com/slideshow/2020-lifestyle-burnout-6012460

National Clinician Guideline Centre (UK). *Patient Experience in Adult NHS Services: Improving the Experience of Care for People Using Adult NHS Services: Patient Experience in Generic Terms.* London: Royal College of Physicians (UK), 2012. https://www.ncbi.nlm.nih.gov/books/NBK115223/

Orsini, Anthony. "Difficult Conversations About Physician Burnout with Dr. Dike Drummond." September 21, 2020. In *Difficult Conversations – Lessons I Learned as an ICU Physician with Dr. Anthony Orsini.* Podcast, MP3 Audio, 40:34. https://theorsiniway.com/podcast-episode-110-dr-dike-drummond/.

Periyakoil, Vyjeyanthi S. "Using Metaphors in Medicine." *The Journal of Palliative Medicine* 11, 6(2008):842-844. https://doi.org/10.1089/jpm.2008.9885

Wilding, Mark, writer. *Grey's Anatomy.* Season 5, episode 6, "Life During Wartime." Directed by James Frawley, featuring Ellen Pompeo, Sandra Oh, and Katherine Heigl. Aired October 30, 2008, on ABC.

Made in the USA
Monee, IL
23 May 2021